Deafness and Challenging Behaviour: The 360° Perspective

Edited by

Sally Austen and Dave Jeffery

Deafness and Challenging Behaviour: The 360° Perspective

Edited by

Sally Austen and Dave Jeffery

John Wiley & Sons, Ltd

Other Wiley Editorial Offices

John Wiley & Sons Inc., 111 River Street, Hoboken, NJ 07030, USA

Jossey-Bass, 989 Market Street, San Francisco, CA 94103-1741, USA

Wiley-VCH Verlag GmbH, Boschstr. 12, D-69469 Weinheim, Germany

John Wiley & Sons Australia Ltd, 42 McDougall Street, Milton, Queensland 4064, Australia

John Wiley & Sons (Asia) Pte Ltd, 2 Clementi Loop #02-01, Jin Xing Distripark, Singapore
129809

John Wily & Sons Canada Ltd, 6045 Freemont Blvd, Mississauga, ONT, L5R 4J3, Canada

Wiley also publishes its books in a variety of electronic formats. Some content that appears
in print may not be available in electronic books.

A catalogue record for this book is available from the British Library

Cloth
ISBN-13   978-0-470-05776-6
ISBN-10   0-470-05776-9

Paper
ISBN-13   978-0-470-02548-2
ISBN-10   0-470-02548-4

Library of Congress Cataloging-in-Publication Data

Deafness and challenging behaviour : the 360 perspective / edited by Sally Austen and
Dave Jeffery.
      p. cm.
   ISBN-13: 978-0-470-05776-6
   ISBN-10: 0-470-05776-9
   ISBN-13: 978-0-470-02548-2
   ISBN-10: 0-470-02548-4
   1. Hearing disorders–Psychological aspects.   2. Deafness–Psychological aspects.
3. Deaf–Mental health.   I. Austen, Sally.   II. Jeffery, Dave.
   RF291.35.D43 2007
   617.8 – dc22
                                                              2007017992

Printed and bound in Great Britain by TJ International Ltd, Padstow, Cornwall
This book is printed on acid-free paper responsibly manufactured from sustainable forestry
in which at least two trees are planted for each one used for paper production.

Dedicated to Ian, with love, on our first anniversary.
Sally

Dedicated to the memory of Naomi King:
a special girl from a special family.
Dave

Contents

Contributors

Sally Austen is a Consultant Clinical Psychologist and has worked with d/Deaf people for over fifteen years. She is employed by Birmingham and Solihull Mental Health Trust and works at Denmark House, National Deaf Mental Health Service, Birmingham.

Di Baines works as a Research Assistant for the Deaf Services at Denmark House, Queen Elizabeth Psychiatric Hospital, Birmingham.

Steve Carney (MB ChB MRCPsych) is currently Consultant Psychiatrist at the National Deaf Mental Health Service and employed by Birmingham and Solihull Mental Health NHS Trust. He previously worked for five years at National Deaf Services in London.

Pat Collins has practised as a nurse in psychiatry for twenty years. For the last eight years, she has been working within Deaf Services, mainly as a community mental health nurse at Denmark House, Birmingham.

Mary Connell, born of Deaf parents, is a near-native user of British Sign Language. She has been a qualified BSL/English Interpreter for twenty years, the past twelve years regularly working in mental health settings. Prior to this, she worked for ten years as a Social Worker with deaf people with a special interest in mental health.

Marian Crowley is a Senior Lecturer at the Department of Community Health and Social Work, University of Central England in Birmingham. She is also a Gestalt Psychotherapist and runs the Gestalt Master's programme at the Sherwood Institute in Nottingham.

Kristyn Eck (MSW LSW) is the Director of Social Services at Columbus Colony Elderly Care in Westerville, Ohio. She obtained her bachelor's degree in Social Work from Rochester Institute of Technology, Rochester, New York in 1997. After graduating with a master's degree in Social Work and a certificate in Gerontology from Syracuse University, New York in 1998, Kristyn began her social work career at CCEC. She has several community projects with an emphasis on improving accessibility to resources and services for deaf older adults in Ohio.

Marlene Eernisse (MS CCC-SLP) is a Speech and Language Pathologist who worked for five years in a residential school for the deaf. She currently works at Bloomington Hospital Children's Therapy Clinic in Bloomington, Indiana.

David M Feldman (PhD) is currently a Psychologist in private practice in Florida, where he is also an Adjunct Professor at the University of Tampa. He recently completed a postdoctoral fellowship in Geropsychology at the University of South Florida and has authored numerous articles on Deafness and Ageing.

Dr Manjit Gahir is a Consultant Forensic Psychiatrist and Lead Consultant of the High Secure Deaf Service at Rampton Hospital in Nottinghamshire. He is also Visiting Reader in the School of Health and Social Care, University of Lincoln.

Dr Alison J Gray is the Consultant Psychiatrist Adviser to the Mental Health Programme of CSIP West Midlands. She was formally Lead Consultant Psychiatrist, National Deaf Mental Health Service, Birmingham.

Adrian Harper is the Communication Officer and Relay Inter-preter at Denmark House, National Deaf Mental Health Service, Birmingham.

Dave Jeffery is a Violence and Personal Safety Specialist Adviser and has worked with Deaf people for ten years. He is currently employed by Birmingham and Solihull Mental Health Trust's Risk Management Department.

Rosie Kentish is a Consultant Child Clinical Psychologist and is cur-rently Head of Child Clinical Psychology at the Nuffield Hearing and Speech Centre at the Royal National Throat, Nose and Ear Hospital in London.

Christine McPherson currently works as Senior Practitioner and Approved Social Worker with National Deaf Mental Health Services, Birmingham and Solihull Mental Health Trust. She is also a quali-fied Psychodynamic Counsellor. She previously worked as Team Leader, Services to Deaf People, Walsall Social Services and has worked with Deaf people for over twenty years.

Dr Sue O'Rourke has worked in mental health and deafness for seventeen years. She is Head of Clinical Psychology at St George

Health Care Group, Manchester providing low secure and open rehabilitation for Deaf people with a forensic history.

Robin Paijmans is a Clinical Psychologist employed by Birmingham and Solihull Mental Health Trust and has worked in community mental health and neuro-rehabilitation. He currently works part-time at Denmark House National Mental Health Services for the Deaf in Birmingham and part-time in cancer care.

Rebecca Reed was a Research Assistant working on the Department of Health, Prison Scoping Exercise: a prison in-reach service for Deaf people.

Judith Vreeland has worked with deaf children and adults as an educator, mental health therapist and programme administrator. She holds a BS in Education of Deaf Children, and an MA in Counselling Deaf Persons. Judy is also trained as a family therapist and completed an advanced programme in organisational leadership through Boston College, in the United States. Judy has been the Director of Walden School, a comprehensive residential treatment centre for deaf children, located in Massachusetts, since 1990.

Leigh Poole Warren (MEd) worked as a School Psychologist with deaf children for four years. Currently, she is teaching a literacy programme with an inner-city school, and is completing work on her doctoral degree.

Preface

Violence and aggression negatively affect service users, staff members and families. People's lives, well-being, health and careers are put at risk. Despite the unequivocal impact of challenging behaviour, little is written about this area, and it seems that resources for dealing with such issues are not forthcoming. The relative prevalence of mental health problems in deaf people is still unclear, but the prevalence of challenging behaviour in deaf people has long been considered greater than in hearing people.

In *Deafness and Challenging Behaviour: The 360° Perspective* contrasting and complementary points of view will cover diagnosis, cause, prevention and management of challenging behaviour in deaf people. Chapters reflect the perspectives of general and forensic psychiatry, learning disability, education, parenting, speech and language therapy, psychology, risk management and therapeutic holding, social work, interpreting, deaf professionals and the criminal justice system. Crucially, the short- and long-term effects on staff working with people who have challenging behaviour is addressed.

This book answers the often asked question: 'How do we manage a deaf person prior to, or at point of, crisis?' It is an obvious question, yet before now its answer has not been readily available. Statutory requirements concerning a systematised approach to the care of those with mental health problems are thwarted by unclear guidance and a lack of recognition of the complexities of working with deaf communities. The pooling of multiple resources within this single volume makes a bold assertion to the traditionally fragmented approach in the care of deaf people with additional needs.

The first chapter of *Deafness and Challenging Behaviour: The 360° Perspective* is written by two service users. It is a frank account that may challenge or disturb the reader but should also inform. It is hoped that its content and honesty will escort and enlighten the reader through the subsequent chapters, which have been written by a wide range of experienced and excellent professional contributors who represent myriad areas of expertise in the field of deafness.

Also to guide later reading, the chapter entitled 'The Anomaly of Deafness' describes the varying deaf-related nomenclature that will be found throughout the book. In order to respect the cultural beliefs of all our contributors, each author has been encouraged to choose and use such terminology as they find appropriate, resulting in consistency of terminology within chapters but not necessarily between chapters. It is acknowledged that challenging behaviour can refer to the 'acting in' behaviours such as eating disorders and self-injury; however, in this book we have deliberately focused on the 'acting out' behaviours such as aggression and violence.

As the editors of *Deafness and Challenging Behaviour: The 360° Perspective*, we particularly wanted to address the contentious issue of physical intervention in the management of aggression and violence in deaf people. Up until now, the lack of knowledge and debate in this area has failed the deaf service user and those who may have to manage challenging behaviour. While this topic remains in its infancy, it is hoped that this book will serve as a foundation from which further research and study will be stimulated.

Despite the breadth of information and number of perspectives covered in this book, one can see the development of an indisputable consensus that **communication** is the key to large parts of the cause, prevention and resolution of challenging behaviour. In writing this book, we were alarmed to realise that, despite this consensus, communication access and language development for deaf people of all ages is still sadly lacking. That deaf children are still being avoidably language-deprived or – delayed is not only tantamount to abuse but also makes the bed that we all must subsequently lie on. Young deaf children, in whose language there has been insufficient investment and whose challenging behaviour is not immediately addressed, will become adults who have challenging behaviour that is more entrenched and harder to manage. Prevention must take precedence over management.

In editing and part writing *Deafness and Challenging Behaviour: The 360° Perspective*, we have learnt an enormous amount from the extremely high standards of work provided by our contributing colleagues. We are extremely grateful for their input. We hope that you enjoy the various chapters as much as we have and that this book will assist you in your continued work with deaf people who have challenging behaviour.

Sally Austen and Dave Jeffery

PART I

Introducing Deafness and Challenging Behaviour

1

The Deaf Service User's Perspective of Challenging Behaviour and Restraint

SALLY AUSTEN AND TWO SERVICE USERS

INTRODUCTION

In this chapter, two ex-service users, both of whom have requested to remain anonymous, describe their life experiences. We are extremely grateful for their help. In order to elicit their views, each was interviewed individually. They were told that this book would include topics such as anger, challenging behaviour and restraint and were asked to describe events that affected them, and their perceptions of them, in their own words. In doing so, each picked themes within this remit that were particularly pertinent to them. They were not asked on this occasion to consider how their actions affected others; and the views of others, which may differ, have not been elicited. Their stories are presented as they were told, with editing only for brevity and flow, without prejudice or censorship, except for reasons of legality or confidentiality. As a result of the lack of censorship, some of the contents may be upsetting to read. This chapter deliberately only represents the views of the service users so that the impact of their experience is not diluted by academic discourse. However, in the discussion some aspects of their narratives are highlighted, and the reader is invited to consider these when reading subsequent chapters of this book.

Deafness and Challenging Behaviour: The 360° Perspective. Edited by S. Austen and D. Jeffery
© 2007 John Wiley & Sons Ltd

SERVICE USER ONE

I was first in a [hearing] psychiatric hospital 20 years ago, and I felt angry many times. The cause of most of my anger was communication problems with the nurses. The first time I was restrained I had been really angry because I was trying to communicate with everyone to explain to them how I was feeling. I got so angry they couldn't understand me that I hit the staff member. Then, all of a sudden, all of these people grabbed me roughly and put me on the floor. I couldn't move my hands, they gave me an injection and then they moved me and put me on a bed. But I don't understand why they were angry with me: I was just trying to communicate with them. Then the next day the doctors came but there was no interpreter and one doctor looked at me and decided that 'This is what you've got' and he whispered to the other doctors. After that they gave me lots of tablets and injections regularly. I thought, 'Why am I taking the tablets and why am I having these injections?' I can remember them walking into the room and tapping me really hard to wake me up and then two nurses forced me to have injections. Eventually, I realised that it must be a regular injection that I had to have every two weeks, but they never explained to me why they were doing this. All they told me was that it was because of my behaviour and that it happens in a lot of hearing psychiatric hospitals.

In the hearing psychiatric hospital I got angry and shouted a lot because there was never an interpreter and there was no communication, which led to problems, and they weren't deaf aware. Then I moved to a deaf psychiatric hospital. I was a bit overwhelmed at first. There were a lot of deaf people there as well as deaf staff and hearing staff that could sign. My signing improved a lot there (I had been brought up poorly, with little education). I learnt to sign, I used an interpreter and I had a communication specialist who taught me to communicate with staff. But I was still very frustrated at what had happened in the past in the hearing hospitals. I was frustrated the way they had treated me, which made me carry on being angry and aggressive to the other staff.

My behaviour escalated: getting angry, fighting staff, getting drunk, setting fires and spending a night in a police cell. I was then moved to a deaf secure facility and it was so much better. I learnt coping skills. I learnt to control myself. I had therapy with a deaf therapist who helped me to express myself. I was able to communicate through the therapy and that meant a lot and really helped. And it helped me move on and be calmer and helped me become better for the future. I was still getting aggressive, but staff would say, 'Control yourself; use the skills you have learnt', and it was much better. I was able to show my emotions. At first, I didn't like that it was a locked hospital. It upset and depressed me but then I realised that they were there to help me; so I accepted it in the end.

And when I was ready I was able to leave to live in a group home with staff support. It was a big difference at first, and for the first year I was up and down – but I never hit staff. I think what helped me change was the communication, and the therapy definitely helped a lot because the therapist was deaf. Now I use more interpreters to access groups in the community. I am a bit disappointed that there aren't more deaf groups, but I have to get on with being confident in the hearing world.

Author: Your first experience of restraint was in a hearing hospital and no one signed and there were no interpreters. Nowadays, it is considered good practice to try to prevent the need for restraint, for example by saying to someone before they are really angry, 'You need to calm down otherwise we will have to restrain you.' How did the hearing hospitals get this message across to you?

They didn't explain anything, as they couldn't sign. They just put me on the floor and injected me and then put me on the bed to sleep it off. It just happened all of a sudden. I had no idea it was going to happen. Several people lay me on my stomach: two held my arms, two held my legs and one sat on my back. It hurt a lot. I had bruises all over my body. My hands and arms and legs and my back all hurt.

Author: What was it like to have someone sitting on your back?

It was difficult to breathe. I was screaming because I couldn't breath properly. I was screaming, 'Get off! Get off! Get off!' but they sat on me for five minutes. But that was 20 years ago. It is better now. They don't sit on your back now.

Author: How did you communicate during the restraint?

I screamed most of the time and tried to communicate. But I couldn't lip-read because I was so upset at being put down on the floor. And I don't think they were trying to talk to me anyway. They were all hearing. And they were all standing up and on top of me so I couldn't see their faces properly anyway. No one was at my level to lip-read.

Author: You said that the first time you were restrained you thought that staff were angry with you. Do you think you might be mistaken, or that they were frightened of you?

No, they were angry with me. I was screaming at staff because they didn't understand my signing; they didn't know what I was saying or why I was angry and so they got angry with me. I could feel it when they restrained me. They weren't frightened of me; they had more power than I did.

Author: Were your experiences different when you were in deaf psychiatric hospital?

First of all, in deaf hospital if I had anxiety and my anger was starting to build up staff would ask if I wanted a one-to-one talk or to go for a walk outside, or ask if I needed PRN tablets [tablets prescribed on a needs basis, to help the person calm down] so maybe I wouldn't get aggressive and I wouldn't need to be restrained.

When I was restrained, it was different. They didn't sit on my back. They would still hold my arms and legs, but I was lying on my back and they would hold my head to turn it so I could see them signing. I was angry at the time; it took a long time to calm down. But it helped as I could see the signing. They kept saying, 'Calm down and in two minutes we will let you go, in two minutes, just calm down first.' So I realised that if I calmed down they would let me go. And so, because of the communication and because I calmed myself down, I didn't need injections. The restraint didn't hurt. And it was completely different because the staff didn't seem angry with me but instead that they were trying to help me.

Author: After deaf psychiatric hospital you went to a deaf secure hospital. Did you experience restraint there?

I was angry a few times and was restrained twice in the two years while I was there. It was different, as they didn't leave you on the floor. They sat you on a chair, which was better, because you were face to face with the interpreter and your chest was free. It was more dignified being sat in a chair than being on the floor. I felt that they respected me more and there were less bruises and nothing hurt like it had on my arms and legs 20 years ago. The other difference is that in the secure hospital they didn't hold my hands. Instead they held my forearms about three inches below my wrist so that I could still move my hands and sign.

Author: You have said a lot about how things improve when there are interpreters, but what about deaf staff or hearing staff that can sign for themselves?

Deaf staff are really good, and some hearing staff are good but they need interpreters. There are usually not many deaf staff, though it is good when there are. Hearing staff, if they can sign, can usually only sign to stage 1 or stage 2 standard. I think there should be more deaf staff and that it would be good if hearing staff could sign for themselves. But the real problem is agency and bank staff as they can't sign at all and who say they want to learn but speak all the time. It is a shame because people get angry when communication is poor.

Author: Have you ever been in a seclusion room?

No, but I have been left in my bedroom after restraint. I felt upset. I was isolated and wanted to talk to someone. They say they leave you on your own to calm down, but I think the better way to help me calm down would be to talk to me. I think it was sometimes an excuse because they couldn't communicate with me.

But in some ways it is good to be moved to the bedroom. There is no privacy during restraint. If it happens where everyone can see, it is awful that others know what staff did. If possible, it would be better to pick the person up and move them to a different place, like the bedroom.

Author: With your experience of challenging behaviour and restraint, how would you want services to improve their care for deaf people with aggression problems?

I have some traumatic memories, especially of being given injections against my will, but things have improved in the last 20 years: from my experience of very rough restraint in hearing hospitals to good communication but restraint on the floor in the deaf psychiatric hospital, and good communication and restraint in a chair in the secure hospital. But there are still lots of things to improve.

- Hearing wards should be taught how to use interpreters and learn how to communicate when patients are upset. They should be trained in deaf awareness and have fire alarms with flashing lights. Also, they should have flashing doorbells on bedroom doors so that staff do not wake you up with a shock by shaking you.

- To help people work on expressing their emotions, and prevent the need for restraint, there should be more therapy with deaf therapists all over the country. Or, if the therapist is hearing, there should be interpreters.
- During restraint, don't sit on a service user's back, as they won't be able to breathe properly.
- During restraint, don't hold a service user's hands (hold their fore-arms instead), as they won't be able to communicate properly. If they are being restrained on the floor, staff should come down to the floor too so that the service user can lip-read or see them signing.
- Where possible, restrain people in chairs so that it is more digni-fied and so that they can see the people with whom they are communicating.

SERVICE USER TWO

I was born the only deaf member of a hearing family. We just used family sign at home. When I went to a deaf oral school where the chil-dren signed among themselves, I was amazed and fascinated that people at school signed properly. I was nervous but wanted to learn. I started to pick up signing at school, but it was very different to at home. It would really frustrate me that I used different signs to people at school. I really wanted to communicate with people, but I wasn't able. I started to feel that my family didn't understand about deafness and communication at all. For example, 'one sleep' was the family sign for 'tomorrow', but at school they had a proper sign for it. When I went home and tried to tell Mum that there was a proper sign for 'tomorrow' she didn't understand and, since I couldn't spell the word, there was no way I could explain. I tried to teach my brother sign but he mostly just used family signing.

Soon after I went to school I was sexually abused. I tried to tell my mother but she didn't understand and I got really frustrated and angry. Mum would say, 'What is the matter with you?' but I had so much anger inside me that I smashed a table and put my hand through the window.

School was really cruel and I got into a lot of trouble. One time I wanted to go to the toilet but the headmaster wouldn't let me. Eventually, I lost control of my bladder. Then I got the cane for weeing myself. It was really annoying, as I couldn't communicate with him. I didn't even know what the word for 'sorry' was. He just kept hitting me. I got really upset and I used to run away to my parents. The abuse happened again and I told them again, but they still didn't understand. I left school at sixteen. They were disappointed with me not staying on to further education, but I thought, 'Stuff school!'

I got into trouble with the police for the first time at a football ground in the 1970s. My team were doing well but needed to win this match. All the supporters seemed to hate the referee. At the last minute, despite the opposition player being offside, the referee allowed the goal. I was so angry I wanted to hit the referee. Lots of people were running onto the pitch. I ran at the referee but the police caught me. I was taken to the police station and questioned, and then taken to court. I was fined five pounds. My parents laughed about it being such a small amount. It was then that my desire to fight the police started.

I didn't want to get involved socially with deaf people, as they weren't getting into trouble. I wanted to hang around with the hearing gangs as they were always fighting. I really enjoyed being part of football violence. I would get excited about kicking people. Sometimes, we would hold someone's head down and then kick it.

On one occasion I was taken to the police station and released without charge after being caught drunk in town trying to break into a shop. On another occasion I went to a football match and then the pub with my girlfriend: she was beautiful and I loved her. There was an altercation starting and a man walking towards my gang so I picked up a bottle, smashed it and lost my head completely. I stabbed him in the face and it took off his nose. As a deterrent, the police said I was no longer allowed to watch home games and had to sign in at the police station during match hours to prove I wasn't at the match. I would still go to the match though: I would go to the police station at the beginning of the game, rush back and climb over the wall to watch the match.

I still enjoyed the football violence. One time, coming out of a match with friends, we joined in a big fight, really kicking people hard and stamping on them. I really enjoyed that. The police came straight away. CID wanted to arrest me and since they had cameras I was sure they had got me this time, but they only moved me on. Later that night, me and some friends started a fight at a disco, pushing past the bouncer so that the hearing gang could get in. Everyone got in and started kicking everything in. The police came and said, 'Oh, it's you again is it?' and sent me home. I didn't go home. I stayed in town and continued to drink.

Finally, after failing to sign in at the police station and getting caught fighting, I was sent to a young person's remand prison for five weeks and then to Crown Court. There was no interpreter so my brother interpreted for me. There were four of us. One was fined £35, the next £30, the next £20 and then it came to me. My brother said, 'I think you are going to prison', and I was really worried. Then I was fined £15! I thought, 'Oh brilliant!' And then the probation officer stood up and said, 'But he broke the terms of his probation order and should go to prison.' The judge said, 'It is too late, I have already made my decision.' So we went out and got drunk and I paid my £15 really easily.

Another phase in my life started when, after stealing some money from a cash register, I was later sent to borstal for a year. But when I left borstal I had been taking a lot of drugs and became very ill. I became moody and paranoid. I was hallucinating that the TV was looking at me, that the devil was coming for me and that I was God. I was only home one night and my parents called the social worker for the deaf who took me to hospital. I was still acting very oddly in hospital and people were scared of me. Eventually, the doctor said I should go to bed but I couldn't understand and didn't know what was going on. So I was put into a wheelchair and given two lots of brown medicine. I fell asleep and woke up in a different hospital.

Over the next few years, I was taken to many different wards and was given injections to make me sleep. But I was in bed all the time and it really hurt because I had bedsores on my ankles and my bottom from being in bed so much. I had strange movements in my legs, which meant that when I was sitting in a chair my heals rubbed themselves sore. I wanted to get up but they kept giving me injections to keep me asleep. Whenever I did get up and walked around, I felt much better, but the nurses kept taking me back to my bed and making me go to sleep. I don't know how many times this happened, maybe 80 or more times. But throughout this I was hallucinating.

Eventually, I did get better and went home to my parents' house, and me and my parents were getting on OK. But then I started getting into trouble again: stealing and fights again.

I was taken to a deaf psychiatric hospital for two weeks but I got into trouble throwing things and drinking alcohol. So the doctor there said that this place wasn't suitable for me and that I had to leave. My parents were really angry that I had to come back home.

After further counts of stealing and fighting, I was sent to a remand prison. There was no communication, just a small hatch to pass food and tablets through. It was so hot. I started to have hallucinations and was moved to hospital. From there, I was taken to court and given bail. When I was bailed I thought, 'Great, I am free. Now I can go out and

fight and do anything I want. I can ignore the court.' That night, I committed theft, arson and seriously assaulted someone. These crimes
ultimately led me to being incarcerated in a secure facility.

In the secure facility and in previous hospitals and prison, I couldn't
communicate with anyone. No one could sign. I didn't know what they
were saying. One time, in a hearing hospital, I signed that I wanted an
interpreter. But the sign for interpreter involves raising the two fingers
of each hand and they thought I was telling them to 'Fuck off' and so
they locked me up. I got a lot of abuse from the staff in prison and in
the secure hospital. It was like a horror story: they would physically
abuse the patients, steal their cigarettes or leave them out in the cold.
The staff didn't like me because I was always fighting them. If they
were restraining me, I couldn't lip-read them as I was on the floor, and
they were holding my hands; so I couldn't sign. But they didn't understand sign; so it made no difference really. But if they were talking and
I couldn't understand them I would just hit them. So then they would
restrain me more. Restraint would really hurt. They would usually get
a cushion and then sit on you. Or kneel on your back. While I was
being restrained, sometimes the men would kick me while I was down
there. I would make sure I saw their faces so I could get them back.
Generally, they would then pick me up and push me to my bedroom
and give me an injection that knocked me out and made me very
confused.

I was in the locked hospital for a long time. I was really angry about
the environment; the fact that they were hearing and there were no
other deaf people or signing people. I got angry, fed up and moody.
The lack of communication made me lose my temper, fight and hit
people. There were ten deaf people in the secure hospital but they were
all spread out and I only had hearing people to communicate with. It
was like living in a horror movie. I would hit my head on the wall or
cut myself really severely until I needed stitches. For about seven years,
I was really rebellious and angry all the time. I tried to hang myself
but a guard found me. I tried to escape but a guard found me and they
kept locking me up. I wanted to be free. My mum begged me to stop
but I didn't.

*Author: So what has changed? How come you are no longer living in
a secure environment?*
Before, when I was small and growing up, nothing changed. And for a
long time in the secure hospital nothing changed. And then in 1987
they came in with an interpreter and a deaf relay interpreter. I didn't

really know what an interpreter was at that time. At that time, my attitude was really bad. The deaf person said in sign language, 'What are you doing? That is stupid. Stop doing that. Stop calling people dick heads.' Then, when I was ready, someone came and we just started talking and it all changed. Life began to change when I first met deaf staff, because of the communication. I hadn't really understood about life and consequently got really angry all the time, swearing and fighting the whole time.

In the secure hospital, they had discussions about things like sex education and the deaf relay made sure that I could understand everything. They started having a discussion about going to the education unit and I thought that I would really like to try education again because this time I would be able to communicate. And they said I could go to a deaf club and thought it would be good for me to talk to people.

It really helped me to start communicating. I can remember a time when I was angry and the interpreter said, 'Look out the window at the weather' and I did and I realised that I didn't want to hit anyone. Once I had interpreters, behaving well was not so boring. I could see the purpose of being good: so that I could go back to education and have interesting conversations.

As my signing improved, so my confidence improved. I was happy. There was still some trouble and communication problems but much less. With interpreters to help, I was like, 'Wow, now I understand! I have been stupid for all this fighting. All the trouble with the police. This is all my fault. And I feel really sorry about it.' And then people in the hospital were happy and I began to improve even more. The fighting finished and I was more natural.

When they said it was time for me to leave the secure hospital, I was so relieved. I went to a deaf rehabilitation facility. I was there for seven years and only in trouble once in that time. Communication was fine because there were interpreters there. To test me, they pulled the interpreters out to see if I would be angry, but I wasn't. I had improved by then and they said I could leave. I had gradual leave to stay with my mother and sister and then I moved to my current staff-supported accommodation and I have not been in any trouble. Now life is better, as I can leave my past behind.

Author: Do you get angry or aggressive now?
I get angry if I see deaf people being teased, but I don't hit out. I walk off. If I am angry now, I have a cup of tea, a smoke or a walk. But here

I can communicate with deaf people and there is no one I need to be suspicious about. Life has really changed now and is calmer.

Author: As you look back on your life, what do think might have made a difference to your behaviour?
The signing. I think if my parents had signed normally that I would be normal. I didn't even know that I was deaf. I didn't know what that meant. I knew that my parents talked and used the phone, but I didn't know what that was and that I was deaf. I thought that as I grew up that I would grow up to talk like them. But then I realised that a boy who was younger than me was talking, and I didn't understand how that worked. But when I went to the deaf school they explained it to me and I was really frustrated. And then not being able to explain the abuse to my parents, when I really wanted to explain it to my mother: that's when I started getting angry.

Author: Children need discipline as they are growing up, to teach them how to behave correctly. Do you think that you had sufficient discipline?
No, definitely not. My parents would tell my sister and brother off and smack them, but wouldn't discipline me at all. I think they thought I was behaving badly just because I was deaf. And they felt sympathy for me because I was deaf. Even if I was angry and started hitting out at people, they reacted with sympathy. I remember once that my father tried to send me to my room in the middle of the day, but my mother said, 'Don't be hard on him. He can't help it – he's deaf.' They knew I got angry quickly and tried to help me control things by saying, 'Don't get angry', but they didn't understand sign language. I think later they shouted at me, but I just ignored it.

Author: When you left school, your behaviour worsened. Your crimes were really quite severe and yet the police interventions, for example fining you or banning you from home matches, do not sound sufficient to prevent your re-offending. Do you think the police and courts were strict enough?
I thought they were strict but, I didn't care what the police said. I **wanted** to get into more trouble. I wanted to be like the hearing gangs. I saw the hearing gangs, how they got into fights and how they were questioned at the police station, and so I knew the way to behave. I just wasn't bothered at the time. But now when I look back I think, 'Oh, you stupid fool.' If the police had punished me more severely from the

start, I don't think it would have deterred me from trouble sooner. I just wasn't bothered. Either way, I would have got into trouble. Because I liked it. It was the same through school, borstal and prison.

Author: You said you liked getting into trouble. What was so good about getting into trouble?
Until I met the interpreters in 1987, behaving well was boring. Behaving well meant having nothing to do. It was silly, but I wanted to do something: break something, fight something. I used to fight a lot at school, and I used to win a lot. A probation officer once offered me the opportunity to learn boxing and I said no. He said, 'Why not? You like fighting.' And I said, 'That's it. I just like fighting.'

Author: How do you look back on your life now?
I wish it had been different. I spent so many years in trouble, and I am sorry about the grief that my trouble caused my family. I was stupid, but I just didn't know. And I am sorry to my mother and father. When this interpreter came into the secure hospital, it just changed. But in some ways it was too late. If I hadn't had these troubles, maybe I would have been married or have had a driving licence by now. Or maybe I would have been free for those 27 years. So I wish it had been different.

I don't hold any resentment or anger for any of the people in my life. No, looking back, I am quite cool. I kind of ignore things now. I am confident and happy. I have staff here who can communicate with me. Before, it was horrible and now it has improved.

Although at times I had two problems, my behaviour and my mental illness, I think my mental illness was because of communication, really because I was so stressed. Now I take a tablet every day and I have an injection every two weeks, but I am not floridly ill at all. And I am content to have the injection.

My parents have both died now. I am not depressed about it. They never really understood me and I never really belonged. I am just happy to be free. I think they are happy too. I think they are looking down on me from wherever they are and they know that my behaviour has improved and are proud of me.

DISCUSSION

The two service users, in part with innocence and in part with insight, lead us to questions that will be addressed in the subsequent chapters of this book.

That both of the narrators ended up in secure accommodation but are now living, trouble free, in open accommodation does beggar questions about service provision, and particularly early intervention. Prior to receiving what they perceived as appropriate services, their challenging behaviour had presumably served a function: perhaps to entertain, control or supply revenge, or perhaps to escape from fear, distress, boredom, confusion or incompetence. As we consider the lifespan of these two individuals, we are challenged to consider whether service provision from cradle to grave has been, or will be, able to provide for their needs or whether service users are expected to mould to the services available.

Both service users identify communication as a cause of their challenging behaviour – either at a specific point in time as a source of frustration or as the very origin of their difficulties in understanding and relating. It is telling that the expectation of the service user is for interpreters and not for deaf staff or hearing staff that sign fluently.

However, the cause of challenging behaviour is likely to be multifactorial. The importance of the 'hearing gang', highly visual role models in a deaf youngster's life, are juxtaposed with a lack of appropriate reinforcement: bad behaviour not being punished, good behaviour so little rewarded that it is perceived as 'boring'. The role of parents, teachers and the criminal justice system as boundary setters is questioned. As with hearing people, diagnosis and risk assessment involves the consideration of behavioural issues alongside the possible presence of mental health problems or cognitive disabilities. If a person exhibits severe challenging behaviour but reveals that for many years they did not know the word 'sorry', diagnosis and issues of culpability are likely to be complex.

These testimonies highlight the perceptions that service users may have (rightly or wrongly) about service providers, for example sometimes perceiving staff as aggressive or angry in response to the service user's aggression. From the specific advice of one of the service users and the narrative of the other, we are drawn to look at the means by which deaf people are restrained, secluded or medicated. From their first-hand experience, the use of accessible therapy, talking, education and fulfilling activity have been recommended as means of preventing and de-escalating aggression.

For these two service users, the beginnings of their stories start more than twenty years ago and both describe improvements in services over time and, perhaps unusually, positive journeys into and then out of secure accommodation. If 'perfect' parenting, education, health and criminal justice services existed, it is still likely that challenging behaviour could not be entirely prevented or eradicated. Furthermore, the responsibility of the individual must be considered alongside the responsibility of others. However, blanket improvements have not occurred. Service users do still die while being restrained, communication in Deaf services provision is not always maximised, deaf mental health patients stay longer in hospital than hearing people and deaf children are still leaving school with disproportionately poor language and social skills. When and how are these situations going to improve?

We are extremely grateful for the help of these two service users.

2

Unravelling the Anomaly of Deafness

DI BAINES

INTRODUCTION

In order to address the issues relevant to challenging behaviour, it was considered necessary to describe the concept of deafness. The aim of this chapter therefore is to provide the reader with an understanding of the complexity and variation of the generic term 'deafness' in order to appreciate the diversities faced within this specialised area. The terminology used to label deafness reflects different perspectives, which encompass aspects of audiometry, communication style, identity and ability and renders a single term untenable. The various classifications of deafness exemplify the need to consider separately the individual's physical, psychological and social experience. They also demonstrate the challenge for service providers. Before exploring the experience of deafness, this chapter will begin by showing the proportion of the population that may fit (albeit sometimes loosely) into such a definition. Finally, a framework for conceptualising deafness is proposed that fits comfortably with the recent World Health Organization (WHO, 2002) recommendations on understanding or describing an individual's personal experience in terms of the degree of functional activity and participation, rather than the old definitions of impairment, handicap and disability (WHO, 1980).

Deafness and Challenging Behaviour: The 360° Perspective. Edited by S. Austen and D. Jeffery
© 2007 John Wiley & Sons Ltd

STATISTICS ON DEAFNESS

The Office for Population Censuses and Surveys, (OPCS, now the Office for National Statistics) Disability Survey found deafness to be the second-most-common disability in the UK (OPCS, 1985). However, there are no definitive *official* figures on deafness, as recognised in the Department of Health's (DoH) paper *Sign of the Times* (DoH, 2002). The latter used the Royal National Institute for Deaf People's (RNID) figures on deafness (whose figures are based on the Medical Research Council's (MRC) Institute of Hearing Research), as opposed to the Office for National Statistics (ONS), which gathers figures from those deaf or hard of hearing people who register with their local social services department. According to the RNID, there are approximately nine million people in the UK who can be described as deaf or hard of hearing, two and a half million of whom are aged between 16 and 60. This suggests that one in eight of the population experience some degree of deafness. There are 698000 people in the UK with severe to profound deafness, 50000–75000 of these being profoundly deaf. In addition, it has been estimated that every year 840 babies in the UK are born with significant deafness (RNID, 2003). It has also been suggested that there may be a higher rate of deafness among certain minority ethnic groups, in particular immigrants to the UK. These higher rates could relate to a variety of factors, including geographical areas where there are greater levels of poverty, inadequate health care, low levels of immunisation against diseases and an acceptance of inter-marriage within certain groups (Ahmad *et al.*, 1998; RNID, 2003).

DEFINITIONS OF DEAFNESS

Deafness does not equate to one single phenomenon but can be defined by various criteria:

- audiometry
- onset of deafness
- identity
- communication style.

AUDIOMETRY

Classically, an individual's deafness has been described in terms of the volume in decibels (dB) required to hear at particular frequencies

Table 2.1 Audiometric measurements and functional capacity

Type of hearing	dBHL	Functional difficulty
Normal hearing	0–20 dBHL	a whisper has an intensity of approximately 15–25 dB and should be audible
Mild deafness	5–39 dBHL	difficulty in following conversational speech especially in noisy environments (a quiet conversation is usually about 30 dB)
Moderate deafness	40–69 dBHL	conversational speech is between 50–65 dB therefore difficulty following speech without hearing aid
Severe deafness	70–94 dBHL	hearing ability limited even with hearing aid (traffic noise is 75–85 dB; noise of hairdryer is 80 dB)
Profound deafness	>95 dBHL	no auditory reception (a pneumatic drill registers at approximately 100 dB, a power lawn mower at 110 dB and a jet plane 35 m away at 140 dB)

(Table 2.1). This is described in terms of the individual's hearing loss (HL) compared to a statistical norm.

Audiometry: the 'Medical Model'

This quantified method of measurement is sometimes interpreted as reflecting the 'medical model of deafness' that conceptualises deafness as a pathological condition or impairment which is disabling and which professionals attempt to treat. In this context, the term 'medical model' is often used pejoratively to imply that the deaf person is reduced only to the functioning of their ears, and that their individuality, opinions or holist functioning are sacrificed to treatment which is imposed on them by oppressive medics (Munoz-Baell and Ruiz, 2000). This demonstrates that there is more to the subjective experience of deafness than can be encompassed in a simple definition of sensory impairment. As such, while the medical model can be usefully explored as an analogy for the experience of being deaf in a hearing world in general, a pejorative use of the term fails to consider that most medics are now aware of a more holistic approach to deafness and do consider social and psychological features alongside physical impairment. It should be noted that the medical model can be implemented by members of any profession (e.g. medics, audiologists, and speech and language therapists).

AGE OF ONSET

Variations in degree of deafness in both ears can vary and make identifying the experience of a hearing loss complicated (Martin, 2001). Furthermore, when consideration is given to other factors such as the age of onset of hearing loss, it could be argued that an audiometric classification, although universally accepted, is overly simplistic. The age of onset of hearing loss has a pervasive effect on language and literacy acquisition and is therefore vital to the understanding of adaptation to deafness (Paul, 1994). There are huge differences environmentally, socially and psychologically between prelingual and postlingual deafness. Kitson and Fry (1990) suggest four different categories of deafness that encompass more of the linguistic and developmental experience of deafness:

1. **Prelingual deafness** (congenital or acquired before language development)
   a) Profound (no speech reception through the ears)
   b) Partial (some difficulty in speech reception)
2. **Postlingual deafness** (acquired after language development)
   a) Profound (no speech reception through the ears)
   b) Partial (some difficulty in speech reception)

Those who become significantly deaf as adults, after having had relatively normal hearing, often describe themselves as 'deafened'. Those who lose part of their hearing in later life, and who compare themselves to their hearing peers, may prefer to use the term 'hard of hearing' or 'hearing impaired' rather than 'partially deaf', even though audiometrically speaking they may have the same hearing thresholds. The variable influencing nomenclature is 'identification'.

IDENTITY

Denmark (1985) argues that prelingual deafness constitutes a sensory deficit, whereas postlingual deafness constitutes a sensory deprivation.

While this explanation may be somewhat black and white, it does provide some explanation for the split definitions of deafness as either a cultural and linguistic lifestyle choice or deafness as a disability. Lane *et al.* (1996) use this categorisation to show how postlingually deafened people tend to mourn a loss of hearing and seek a cure, whereas deaf people see themselves as a distinct linguistic and cultural group that seek recognition and acceptance rather than 'fixing'.

The use of a lower-case 'd' tends to be used either to refer to the audiological state of being deaf or when referring to those who do not use sign language, those who may regard their deafness as a disability and those who socialise generally within the hearing population. For example, an elderly hearing person who has lost their hearing naturally as a result of ageing would be unlikely to learn sign language or become a member of the Deaf community. In addition, some partially deaf or hearing-impaired people feel they are caught between two worlds, the hearing and the Deaf, and don't feel they fit comfortably in either (Woodcock and Aguayo, 2000).

Deaf Culture

Deaf people who adhere to the Deaf culture regard themselves as an exclusive minority group that developed from a resistance to assimilate into a hearing society and to create a positive identity (Ahmad *et al.*, 1998). Central to membership of the Deaf community is the use of sign language. Deaf culture encompasses not just a unique form of communication but also a social protocol, providing a sense of belonging, pride and support. Baker and Padden (1978) describe this as 'attitudinal deafness'. In families where deafness runs congenitally there tends to be a much stronger identification with Deaf culture; however, the majority of deaf people are born into hearing families and many members of the Deaf community only become aware of a 'different' approach to their deafness when attending residential schools.

The two cornerstones of the Deaf community are Deaf residential schools and Deaf clubs. The latter providing interaction and participation with community members across generations and enabling members to transcend the negative experiences of daily interaction within a hearing society and create the ability to obtain political strength to lobby the larger community (Meadow-Orlans and Erting, 2000). Geographically, Deaf people are widely dispersed and Deaf clubs provide a central meeting place where Deaf people can share news, information and entertainment using a shared, natural language. However, in recent years with the introduction of new technology, such as email, Internet chatrooms and mobile text messaging, it is felt that patterns of socialisation are changing among young Deaf people and attendance at Deaf clubs has decreased (Austen, 2004).

COMMUNICATION

The variation in methods of communication adopted by deaf people is complex. Communication methods of deaf people vary according to:

- type and degree of deafness
- age of onset
- cognitive abilities
- language skills
- geographical area and availability of various types of communication
- type of schooling
- the sociopolitical climate of the time
- audiological status and identity choice of the individual's parents
- presence or absence of Deaf role models
- subjective views of the individual, their family and their audiological/educational advisers.

British Sign Language (BSL) is a fully functional and expressive language that developed over hundreds of years by Deaf people using hand shapes, facial expression, gestures and body language to convey meaning (as are most native sign languages). It is not a visual representation of spoken language but follows its own unique set of grammatical rules and structure. On 18 March 2003 the UK government formally recognised BSL as an official language. There are roughly 50 000 people in the UK whose first language is BSL (RNID, 2003).

Sign language use (manual communication) is broadly associated with earlier and more profound deafness and with additional language or cognitive difficulties. Milder and later-onset deafness tends be linked with oral communication. Oral communication may involve maximising the use of residual hearing by using assistive aids such as hearing aids or cochlear implants (Acker and Crocker, 2004), lip-reading, speech and written communication.

The focus on communication as either being oral or manual distracts from the crucial fact that many deaf people from impoverished language backgrounds may have little formal language at all. Language that is limited to some home signs (signs that are not widely understood outside of the immediate social grouping), gestures and the writing of a few words are not sufficient for independent functioning, and deaf people with minimal language skills, who may also have been raised in social isolation, often require support from mental health or social services (du Feu and Fergusson, 2003).

The 'Oral–Manual debate' (Austen and Coleman, 2004) describes an historic and ongoing disagreement between the proponents of either signed or oral communication, particularly in education. Neisser (1983) considers speech an unrealistic goal for Deaf people:

> The hearing world is deeply biased toward its own oral language, and always prefers to deal with deaf people who can speak. But speech is always difficult for the deaf, never natural, never automatic, never without stress. It violates their integrity, they have a deep biological bias for the language of signs. (Neisser, 1983, p. 281)

However, where the two styles were seen as mutually exclusive there are now positive results coming from their marriage. For example, some cochlear implant departments now insist on implantees learning sign language pre- and post-implant so that their language skills can be improving while waiting for the audiological benefits of the implant to be seen (Crocker, 2005, personal communication).

EXPERIENCE OF DEAFNESS

Alongside the varying definitions of deafness are a number of variables that can influence the individuals' experience of deafness. These are:

- parentage
- schooling
- functional ability
- cause of deafness and additional disabilities
- access to services
- experience of stigma.

PARENTAGE: AUDIOLOGICAL STATUS AND IDENTITY

It is important to recognise and understand how social, environmental and cultural factors can impact greatly on life experiences both negatively and positively. For example, a deaf child with hearing parents will have very different life experiences than a Deaf child with Deaf parents. The majority of deaf children are born to hearing parents and therefore are born into an intimate setting of difference; difficulties begin with access to the language and communication system of parents. Parents' perception and reaction to their child's deafness can impact greatly on the emotional, social, educational and vocational development of a child both positively and negatively (Sands and Crocker, 2004).

Hearing parents may be more likely to perceive their child's deafness as a tragedy and feel poorly equipped to cope with parenting a deaf child. Deaf parents of Deaf children may feel more equipped and have more positive experiences of deafness than their hearing counterparts. There is evidence that, as a result of positive language and social role models, Deaf children of Deaf parents have mental health, language development and behaviour that is better than deaf children of hearing parents and equal to that of hearing children (Paul and Quigley, 1990; Meadow-Orlans, 1990). In addition, Deaf children of Deaf parents tend to have fewer additional disabilities, as their cause of deafness is less likely to be traumatic.

TYPE OF SCHOOLING

One major factor of the experience of deafness is that of the delivery of education. The historic negative perception of deafness, i.e. the 'deaf and dumb' label, resulted in the late arrival of deaf schools into the education arena. In addition, owing to their scarcity and geographic location, the majority of these 'special' schools were, and still are, boarding schools.

The question as to appropriate methods of communication with and delivery of education to deaf children, i.e. oral or manual, was hotly debated during the late-nineteenth and twentieth centuries. Prominent oralists, such as Alexander Graham Bell, insisted that deaf children should be taught to communicate solely by lip-reading, speaking and writing; manual supporters argued that sign language was both beneficial and vital to communication for deaf people (Meath-Lang,1996). The debate reached its climax at the famous (although some would argue rather controversial) international conference in Milan in 1880 (Moore and Levitan, 1993). The outcome of the conference was to govern the way in which deaf children would be educated for decades to come. Education was considered best delivered in an oral environment where deaf children, regardless of the degree of deafness, would be forbidden to sign.

However, despite attempts to suppress the use of sign language in schools during this period, signing in schools essentially went underground, continuing (in secret) outside of the classrooms, which ensured the continuity of Deaf language and culture. Although this type of education may have benefited some deaf children in their ability to communicate orally, it was eventually recognised that for many profoundly deaf children this system of education was of little or no use to them and resulted only in frustration and poor academic achievement. In recent years with sign language now recognised as an official language, methods of teaching are beginning to (although not wholly) move back towards a more manual approach. In addition, with the emphasis in recent years on the inclusion and integration of diversities into mainstream schools, there has been a growing number of deaf children educated in local schools. It could be argued that there are both positive and negative aspects to localised education: positive in relation to the avoidance of any emotional detachment from the family unit that could be associated with residential education and also an increased level of social and academic parental involvement, and negative in relation to a denial of contact/identity with deaf peers and therefore language and culture, and the danger of a sense of isolation associated with **generally** being the only representative of a minority group.

FUNCTIONAL ABILITY

Profoundly deaf people are considered disabled when compared to the hearing norm, owing to their inability to hear. It is argued, however, that the extent an inability to hear is considered 'disabling' depends largely on whether the deafness has been embraced as a pathology or as a difference. Culturally, Deaf people have acquired a complete language and therefore are able to communicate fully within the Deaf community. Their limitation in communication is only demonstrated when trying to communicate within a hearing world. However, if access to appropriate technology is available together with positive societal attitudes (Deaf awareness), the barrier to communication can be minimal. On the other hand, the functional ability of a deaf individual without the capacity to fully communicate within either a deaf or hearing population is far more disabling. The latter would include individuals who experienced late-onset deafness, or deaf individuals who have been denied access to any appropriate communication mode or due to additional disabling conditions that may impede acquisition of any useful communication.

CAUSE OF DEAFNESS AND ADDITIONAL DISABILITY

Deaf people presenting to clinicians can often have a variety of additional impairments that can make providing the necessary response and treatment more complicated. The majority of prelingually profoundly deaf people are born to hearing parents and therefore their deafness is not as a result of genetic inheritance but rather as a result of external factors, e.g. prematurity, maternal illness such as rubella, or early childhood illness such as meningitis. For this reason, many deaf people have additional impairments, e.g. cardiac, visual or learning disabilities. Crocker and Edwards (2004) estimate that 40% of deaf children have additional disabilities. It has been reported that approximately 15% of people deafened by meningitis have associated learning disabilities (Freeman *et al.*, 1981) and similarly recent statistics have identified 23 000 deaf-blind people living in the UK (RNID, 2003).

ACCESS TO SERVICES

In many developed countries in recent decades, a legal obligation has been placed on all service providers whether in relation to health, education, social services or employment, to address the needs of individuals with disabilities, which include the deaf. However, different regional interpretations of legislation together with different levels of understanding/awareness of needs and financial constraints have led to huge variations in the quality and quantity of service provision and access to those services. For example, the UK's Disability Discrimination Act requires service providers to make 'reasonable adjustments' to ensure accessibility to services. A basic reasonable adjustment to enable a deaf individual to gain initial access to a service could arguably be to provide an interpreter. However, with a recognised national shortage of sign language interpreters in the UK and elsewhere, a lack of knowledge as to the process of booking an interpreter and the cost of hiring the same, the provision of an interpreter very often does not convert well into reality. In these situations, especially in primary health care and social services, family members (often children) are brought in to act as interpreters, which, in a medical context, could be considered highly controversial giving rise to issues of confidentiality, misrepresentation and the danger of misdiagnosis.

It could be argued that investment in modern technology (e.g. relay services, video conferencing etc.) could go some way in addressing this problem, but very often this is dependent on an individual's intuition and response (e.g. a sympathetic GP) rather than a universal insistence.

It could be argued therefore that deaf people, despite legislative moves, are still at greater risk than their hearing peers of experiencing more severe and complex health problems, both mental and physical, because of problems related to early intervention, diagnosis and primary care.

The barriers to deaf people accessing services are not necessarily restricted to the practical difficulties related to the provision of services. Negative perceptions towards mental health services within the Deaf community that originate from the historical misunderstanding and treatment of the deaf (e.g. deaf people being placed in mental hospitals solely for their deafness) often result in an avoidance to seek help. This was demonstrated in a study by Steinberg *et al.* (1998) where Deaf participants used signs such as 'prison', 'straitjacket', or 'crazy house' when referring to mental hospitals.

Where specialist services are available, owing to their scarcity, it is very often geographical logistics that govern a positive or negative experience of access. The difficulties in accessing services that have been shown to magnify mental health problems (du Feu and Fergusson, 2003) are further exacerbated by a lack of rehabilitation facilities. A recent study at a specialist mental health unit for the Deaf in the UK suggests that a lack of appropriate community rehabilitation facilities very often governs the length of hospital stay of mental health patients more than health factors. The average length of hospital stay for deaf patients was shown to be statistically double that of their hearing peers (Patterson and Baines, 2005).

It is important to note, however, that access to services is not homogeneous and is dependent on many factors, some of which have been discussed above. Localised access to hospitals and GPs who adopt good standards of practice with regard to Deaf awareness, local education facilities and access to local Deaf clubs to name just a few, can and do ensure positive experiences for many deaf people.

EXPERIENCE OF STIGMATISATION AND OPPRESSION

Historically, deaf people have been perceived and treated negatively. The term 'deaf and dumb' came from a belief that the inability to communicate orally equated to an inability to think (Higgins, 1980). Although it could be argued that the term 'dumb' merely describes an inability to speak, it could similarly be interpreted as implying that deaf people are inferior and stupid. The latter perception led to many deaf people being placed in asylums or institutional care with no formal diagnosis (Denmark, 1985, 1994). Further examples of negative assumptions and oppression can be traced back in history. During Roman times, deaf people were denied any legal rights; during the Middle Ages, it was believed that an inability to speak the sacraments denied deaf people immortality; during the 1800s, deaf people in America were denied the right to vote, and many American states forbade deaf people from making contracts (Higgins, 1980). Moving on through to the late-nineteenth century, further examples of oppression are the banning of sign language in schools and the extreme example of racial cleansing in Nazi Germany between 1933 and 1945 that led first to the sterilisation of 17000 deaf people and eventually to the slaughter of thousands (Biesold, 1999).

Oppression and stigmatisation are generally seen, or at least often only considered, as being part of the experience of the profoundly deaf. However, consideration should also be given to the stigmatisation of those with partial deafness/hard of hearing. McCay and Andrews (1990) suggest that due to poor educational achievement, problems with communication and employer attitudes the occupational level of this group is significantly lower than that of the hearing population. Levels of unemployment have also been found to be higher among the partial hard-of-hearing population. This is also the case with profoundly deaf people. In 1999, a RNID survey showed that deaf people had an unemployment rate that was four times the national average and that those in work had an average income of under £10000 p.a. (RNID, 2003). Similar findings have been reported in the USA.

CONCEPTUALISING DEAFNESS: THE PAIJMAN–BAINES MODEL

Whereas the Disability Discrimination Act 1995 placed a legal definition on deafness as a disability using a hearing norm; the World Health Organization (WHO, 2002) recently adopted a more holistic approach considering an individual's experience within the context of functions, structures, activity and participation. The *International Classification of Impairments, Disabilities and Handicaps*, 1980 (ICIDH) (WHO, 1980) was replaced in 2002 by the *International Classification of Functioning, Disability and Health* (ICF) (WHO, 2002). The ICF was intended to be a more universal approach to physical and mental impairments. In the case of deafness, this could arguably help to identify the cultural and social differences of experience. With this in mind a framework to conceptualise deafness that attempts to identify the variation in factors that govern perception, experience and socialisation of the condition, both positive and negative, is suggested. However, as with any framework, it is important to note that there is always the danger of oversimplification. Essentially, this framework works on the assumption that a late-onset deafened person may be more likely to conceptualise things from a 'hearing world' perspective and a congenitally deaf person more likely to conceptualise things from a 'Deaf world' perspective. Thus, the need to consider variations that may not necessarily fit well within the framework is necessary. For example, there are some congenitally deaf people who will still conceptualise their deafness as an impairment and disability, and do not identify with Deaf culture at all; whereas some late-onset deafened people will negotiate their journey of adjustment to come to identify with and live in the Deaf world. Each person's path of adjustment is different. Therefore, it is important to consider a possible juxtaposition between the 'deaf world' and the 'hearing world' that overlap with each other. Nevertheless, the framework suggests deafness to be viewed on a continuum with deafness as a 'condition' at one end and deafness as an 'identity' at the other. Between these two quite different perspectives

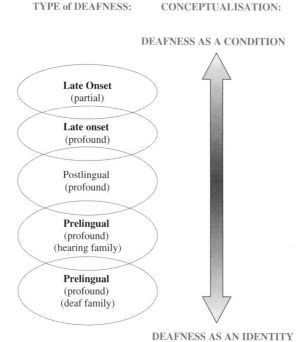

Figure 2.1 The Paijmans–Baines model (Paijmans and Baines, in preparation)

are factors and considerations, which have been discussed during the course of the chapter, that will impact on the experience of deafness.

CONCLUSION

In trying to understand deafness we try to create norms with which to compare and contrast. It is often argued that using hearing as the norm by which to examine deafness is inappropriate, as it misses or betrays the cultural difference of deaf people and the deaf experience. In this chapter, we have demonstrated that the problem may not be the use of a hearing norm but the assumption that there is a deaf norm that requires examining. The group that is so flippantly referred to as 'deaf' is actually a patchwork of people with such wide-ranging physical, psychological and social experiences that any definition of deafness is virtually arbitrary.

In this context, it should be recognised that to empathise clinically with a deaf individual or to identify a research cohort essentially requires the acquisition of a basic understanding of the whole experience of deafness, i.e. cultural, social and psychological. Finally, a framework conceptualising deafness has been suggested that in essence brings together many aspects of experience discussed throughout the chapter which may go some way to identifying such an experience. However, it could be argued that even this could be construed as an oversimplification of a very complex phenomenon.

REFERENCES

Acker T, Crocker S (2004) Tip-toeing through technology. In Austen S, Crocker S (eds), *Deafness in Mind: Working Psychologically with Deaf People Across the Lifespan*, London, Whurr, pp. 53–72.

Ahmad W, Darr A, Jones L, Nisar G (1998) *Deafness and Ethnicity: Service, Policy and Politics*, Bristol, The Policy Press.

Austen S (2004) Older Adults who use sign language. In Austen S, Crocker S (eds), *Deafness in Mind: Working Psychologically Across the Lifespan*, London, Whurr, pp. 329–44.

Austen S, Coleman E (2004) Controversy in deafness: *Animal Farm* meets *Brave New World*. In Austen S, Crocker S (eds), *Deafness in Mind: Working Psychologically with Deaf People Across the Lifespan*, London, Whurr, pp. 3–20.

Baker C, Padden C (1978) *American Sign Language: A Look at its History, Structure and Community*, Silver Spring, Linstok Press.

Biesold H (1999) *Crying Hands: Eugenics and Deaf People in Nazi Germany*, Washington, Gallaudet University Press.

Crocker S, Edwards L (2004) Deafness and additional difficulties. In Austen S, Crocker S (eds), *Deafness in Mind: Working Psychologically with Deaf People Across the Lifespan*, London, Whurr, pp. 252–69.

Denmark JC (1985) A study of 250 patients referred to a department of psychiatry for the deaf. *British Journal of Psychiatry* 146(March): 282–6.

Denmark JC (1994) *Deafness and Mental Health*, London, Jessica Kingsley.

Department of Health (2002) *A Sign of the Times: Modernising Mental Health Services for People Who are Deaf*, London, Department of Health.

du Feu M, Fergusson K (2003) Sensory impairment and mental health. *Advances in Psychiatric Treatment* 9: 95–103.

Freeman RD, Carbin CF, Boese RJ (1981) *Can't Your Child Hear? A Guide for Those Who Care about Deaf children*, Croom, Helm.

Higgins C (1980) *Outsiders in a Hearing World: A Sociology of Deafness*, London, SAGE.

Kitson N, Fry R (1990) Prelingual deafness and psychiatry. *British Journal of Hospital Medicine* 44(5): 353–6.

Lane H, Hoffmeister R, Bahan B (1996) *A Journey into the Deaf-World*, San Diego, Dawn Sign Press.

Martin M (2001) Deaf and hard of hearing people. In Graham J, Martin M (eds), *Ballantyne's Deafness* (6th edn.), London, Whurr, pp. 1–9.

McCay V, Andrews JF (1990) *The Psychology of Deafness: Understanding Deaf and Hard of Hearing People*, New York, Longman.

Meadow-Orlans K (1990) Research on developmental aspects of deafness. In Moores D, Meadow-Orlans K (eds), *Educational and Developmental Aspects of Deafness*, Washington, Gallaudet University Press, pp. 283–98.

Meadow-Orlans K, Erting C (2000) Deaf people in society. In Hindley P, Kitson N (eds), *Mental Health and Deafness*, London, Whurr, pp. 3–24.

Meath-Lang B (1996) Cultural and language diversity in the curriculum: toward reflective practice. In Parasnis I (ed), *Cultural and Language Diversity and the Deaf Experience*, Cambridge, Cambridge University Press, pp. 160–70.

Moore MS, Levitan L (1993) *For Hearing People Only*, Rochester, NY, MSM Productions.

Munoz-Baell IM, Ruiz MT (2000) Empowering the deaf: let the deaf be deaf. *Journal of Epidemiology and Community Health* 54(1): 40–4.

Neisser A (1983) *The Other Side of Silence: Sign Language and the Deaf Community in America*, New York: Alfred A Knopf.

Office of Population Censuses and Statistics (1985) *The Prevalence of Disability Among Adults*, London, HMSO.

Paijmans R, Baines D (in preparation) Impairment or identity: a framework for conceptualising deafness and assessing its psychological impact.

Patterson N, Baines D (2005) The Psychosocial influences affecting the length of hospital stay of Deaf mental Health service users. 3rd Mental Health and Deafness World Conference 2005, Worcester, South Africa, 26–29 October 2005.

Paul PV (1994) *Language and Deafness* (2nd edn.), San Diego, Singular Publishing Group.

Paul PV, Quigley SP (1990) *Education and Deafness*, New York, Longman.

RNID (2003) *Facts and Figures on Deafness and Tinnitus*, London, Royal National Institute for Deaf People.

Sands E, Crocker S (2004) Paediatric cochlear implantation. In Austen S, Crocker S (eds), *Deafness in Mind: Working Psychologically with Deaf People Across the Lifespan*, London, Whurr, pp. 235–51.

Steinberg AG, Sullivan VJ, Loew RC (1998) Cultural and linguistic barriers to mental health service access: the deaf consumer's perspective. *American Journal of Psychiatry* 155(7): 982–4.

World Health Organization (1980) *World Health Organization: International Classification of Impairments, Disabilities and Handicaps*, Geneva, World Health Organization.

World Health Organization (2002) *International Classification of Functioning, Disability and Health (ICF)*, Geneva, World Health Organization.

Woodcock K, Aguayo M (2000) *Deafened People: Adjustment and Support*, London, The University of Toronto Press.

3

Bearing Witness: Challenging Behaviour and its Contribution to Trauma and Vicarious Trauma

DAVE JEFFERY, MARIAN CROWLEY AND SALLY AUSTEN

INTRODUCTION

The mental health professional (MHP) is exposed to high levels of trauma during the course of their work. Moreover, the main cause of stress experienced by MHPs is violence and aggression perpetrated by service users (National Audit Office, 2003). Staff can be traumatised by being the direct recipients of violence or threatened violence. However, witnessing violence aimed at others and receiving information about the traumatisation of others can also traumatise staff vicariously. Recent research published by the Healthcare Commission (HC) has established that 89% of MHPs in the UK have witnessed incidents of assault, with a further 75% having been the victim of physical or verbal assault (HC, 2005).

This chapter explores the contribution of challenging behaviour to trauma and vicarious trauma (VT). It is intended to stimulate discussion and highlight the importance for further research in this area. Narratives illustrate the experience of individuals working with service users exhibiting challenging behaviour or who are traumatised themselves. These experiences will be used to indicate positive practice or

Deafness and Challenging Behaviour: The 360° Perspective. Edited by S. Austen and D. Jeffery
© 2007 John Wiley & Sons Ltd

areas of deficit within organisational systems. The authors offer suggestions to bridge current gaps in service provision. It is argued that lack of appropriate support for staff that have experienced trauma or VT can result in less effective risk assessment and de-escalation, which in turn increases the prevalence of challenging behaviour. The chapter is aimed at all MHPs working with, or exposed to, challenging behaviour. While some elements may relate to specific disciplines, the overall themes can be readily transferred to generalised care staff, settings and environments.

Little has been written about the experience of trauma or VT in deaf staff or staff working with deaf service users. However, it is hypothesised that deaf staff and sign language interpreters may be more vulnerable to VT for reasons to do with their cultural, linguistic and emotional proximity to their service users. It is also hypothesised that the visual nature of sign language can increase the listener's (receiver's) vulnerability to VT. It is argued that deaf staff and sign language interpreters are less likely than hearing staff to receive the support and supervision that have proved to be protective factors from trauma and VT.

TRAUMA

The word 'trauma' is derived from the Greek word *trauma* meaning a wound (Merriam-Webster, 2003). Freud looked at psychological trauma when he was studying the cause of hysteria and referred to the impact of not having a place of safety outside or within to withdraw into at times of dread (Freud, 1959). The American Psychiatric Association (APA) *Diagnostic and Statistical Manual* (APA, 2000) discusses trauma when referring to post-traumatic stress disorder (PTSD). In this context, the person is considered to have PTSD if certain diagnostic factors are in evidence and the antecedent experience involves:

> the person experienced, witnessed or was confronted with an event . . . and the person's response involved intense fear or helplessness (APA, 2000, pp. 427–28).

Furthermore, Pearlman and Saakvitne (1995) explore trauma from a constructivist self-development standpoint in which parts of the self are impacted by the trauma. As a consequence of the trauma, an individual's basic assumptions, or beliefs about themselves and the world, are often challenged (Pearlman and MacIan, 1995). It is important to acknowledge that, just as trauma impacts and changes our service user's hearing (or receiving in sign language), traumatic material impacts on the listener's own sense of self. Pearlman and Saakvitne (1995) point out that 'these alterations include shifts in the therapist's identity and world view' (p. 152).

The uniqueness of an individual's response to trauma is determined by the meaning they ascribe to it, their experience and understanding of themselves, their emotional, psychological and interpersonal experiences and their environment (Pearlman and MacIan, 1995). Trauma can therefore be defined by the experience of the individual: it is their subjective experience that determines whether an event is or is not traumatic (Allen, 1995). While each individual staff member will perceive an event uniquely, it is also likely that groups that share similar life experiences, e.g. deaf staff members or interpreters may differ from hearing staff members as a group who will not have had those same experiences.

VICARIOUS TRAUMA

Over the past two decades, differing terms have been used to describe the effects of working with others who experience trauma. McCann and Pearlman (1990) refer to it as vicarious traumatisation (VT). Other writers have coined their own terms when referring to this phenomena, e.g. 'compassion fatigue' (Figley, 1995), 'secondary traumatic stress disorder' (Munroe *et al.*, 1995) and 'traumatic countertransference' (Herman, 1992). VT is a relatively new and unexplored construct, a process that involves psychic contamination, whereby the service user's emotional experience intrudes into our unconscious, in many instances without our being aware of it.

The literature identifies that counsellors, psychotherapists and other MHPs, despite being trained to work with service users presenting with varying degrees of emotional and psychological issues, are faced with additional challenges when working with service users who have experienced trauma. Furthermore, McCann and Pearlman (1990) would argue that VT is inevitable if you're going to work with trauma. Pearlman and Saakvitne (1995) define VT as 'the transformation that occurs in the inner experience of the therapist [or worker] that comes about as a result of empathic engagement with a service user's trauma material' (p. 31). As a consequence of our work with service users, disruption to one's beliefs and intrusive imagery is possible:

nightmares, fear about one's own safety, questioning one's own life experiences and vulnerabilities may occur.

Figely (1995) points out that MHPs can be traumatised without actually being physically harmed; simply hearing about a traumatic event can traumatise them. This would equate to a deaf person or an MHP who works with deaf service users being informed about a traumatic event in sign language. In sign language, this could be more traumatising than in speech. The visual nature of sign language involves iconic signs and mime. As such, more information and detail of the event is expressed in sign than in the equivalent spoken account. The degree of violence, power and powerlessness, pain, fear and speed would all be etched on the faces, hands and body language of the person recounting the story. Furthermore, whereas the traumatic spoken narrative would only be retained in the verbal memory, the signed narrative is retained in both the visual and verbal (linguistic) memories of the receiver. For the sign language interpreter and deaf relay interpreter, the traumatic imagery has to be processed and translated in such detail and with such vivid understanding of the narrative that there is no possibility of personal denial. For example, the spoken English phrase 'I was hit' can be understood without the need for any other information. However, to be able to translate the phrase into sign language, making use of three-dimensional directional verbs and non-manual features such as body language and facial expression, the interpreter must process unspoken information or request further spoken information. In the process of doing their job properly, they will open themselves up to further traumatic material. Harvey (2001) highlights the fact that sign language interpreters may experience vicarious emotional trauma working in clinical settings.

Empathetic identification may be one of the factors that lead people to choose the role of helper. Furthermore, it has been identified among those who have immense capacity for feeling and expressing empathy that they tend to be more at risk of VT (Figley, 1995). Although there is no current research, it would be fair to hypothesise that deaf staff members empathise more with deaf service users who have traumatic experiences than hearing staff with deaf services users or deaf staff with hearing service users. Empathy tends to increase with the number of shared experiences. The Deaf world is remarkably small, with only 50–70000 sign language users in the UK (British Deaf Association, 1999), and deaf people have commonly been educated in specialist deaf schools. There is a high likelihood that some deaf staff will have been to school with deaf service users or will know them socially outside of the clinical environment. For hearing MHPs, this tends only to happen with those who live within the catchment area of their workplace. The deaf person's social and educational experiences tend to be conducted over a much wider geographic range, if not nationally. MHPs need to be aware that they may be changed by the impact of listening to the service user's experience. It's important to note that MHPs' reactions, unless understood and brought into awareness, may lead to disruptions to the therapeutic relationship.

COUNTERTRANSFERENCE

Friedman (1997) asserts that countertransference is more likely to occur when a service user's history triggers memories in the MHP. In countertransference, the therapist's own unresolved unconscious feelings and conflicts are activated. Countertransference reactions in MHPs can provide a valuable insight into the emotional world of the service user.

Herman (1997) points out that 'traumatic counter-transference . . . occurs when the therapist experiences, to a lesser degree, the same terror, rage and despair as the patient' and that 'the patient's story is bound to revive personal traumatic experiences that the therapist may have suffered' (p. 40).

Although separated by the patient/service user status, deaf staff may share many difficult life experiences with deaf service users. Whether service user or staff, deaf people are often discriminated against, oppressed or teased, often by hearing people (RNID, 1998). They are more likely to have been sexually abused, usually by hearing people (Sullivan *et al.*, 2000) and to be in low-paid jobs and have few academic qualifications (McCay and Andrews, 1990). In recounting their history, or their perceptions of the cause of their difficulties, the deaf service user is likely to remind the deaf staff member of many of their own difficulties. In a deaf service it is likely that most of the staff will still be hearing, better qualified and better paid than the deaf staff. There may well be communication oppression (with spoken language taking precedence over sign language). Thus, the negative experiences of both the deaf service user and the deaf staff member are not just narratives of the past but are happening currently. For those interpreters who are hearing children of deaf adults, an overidentification with the deaf service user and strong reactions to issues raised in therapy may occur (Napier and Cornes, 2004).

THE RELATIONSHIP BETWEEN TRAUMA AND CHALLENGING BEHAVIOUR

Research has indicated that there is an association between violence and aggression as an expression of trauma (Bloom and Reichert, 1998). McSwain *et al.* (1998) note that MHPs are exposed to trauma in that they listen to service users' experiences and bear witness to the expression of emotional pain in the form of aggression, hostility and acts of self-harm and suicide.

What is clear is that maladaptive coping strategies are an attempt to resolve a person's inner pain. The outcome is the paradox that the person's 'solutions' (challenging behaviour) invariably become the care staff's 'problem' (managing challenging behaviour). This will be the same whether in deaf or hearing services, and whether referring to deaf or hearing staff.

It is the human condition to protect oneself from harm. The use of a biological response to an emotional trigger is the legacy of our ancestors' basic need for survival as a species. Termed 'fight or flight' (Horowitz, 1986), this process reflects the two fundamental choices open to those who are presented with a dangerous situation. For those providing care to individuals who demonstrate challenging behaviour, natural instincts have to be countered since the act of caring in modern society is informed by legal, professional and ethical paradigms and not primordial instinct and intuition.

With each exposure to the fight-or-flight process the psyche remembers and makes associations with the experience or event that triggers it. MHPs exposed to repeat incidents of violence (either as a victim or a witness) will have the potential to accumulate and ascribe posthumous value to current emotional events (Bloom and Reichert, 1998). There is a consequent argument that to effectively manage challenging behaviour an emotional middle ground needs to be found, otherwise fight or flight will continue to dictate our response to crisis events.

THE IMPACT OF CHALLENGING BEHAVIOUR: CASE EXAMPLES

Using a narrative format, the following case examples give subjective accounts of the professionals' experiences of working with challenging behaviour. It has been suggested that a person's narrative is a viable tool in establishing emergent emotional themes (Barker, 2002).

The important value of the narrative is the concept of re-empowering the person. This is of primary significance given the feelings of powerlessness that influence individuals who suffer with PTSD. There is also an added facet concerning the narrative informing the supportive process. The person will need to find resolution and not solely rely upon prophylactic treatment. This can be illustrated by the observations of Barker and Buchanan-Barker:

> By offering (and especially by imposing) diagnosis, which people have not asked for, we disempower them by subjecting their original story, and invalidating all the lived experience associated with it. (Barker and Buchanan-Barker, 2004, p. 19)

Case Study One

I was working on an intensive care unit several years ago and one service user was becoming increasingly more agitated and delusional as the morning progressed. I reported this to senior staff but felt that my concerns were being ignored. To cut a long story short, the service user walked up to me and grabbed my shirt below my throat and said, 'I'm going to kill you.' Other members of staff managed to restrain him before he could land a blow with a fist three times the size of my own.

After the event, I went about my duties, filled in the incident reports and completed my shift. When I got to my car, I began to shake uncontrollably and could not get the face of the service user out of my mind. That night I could not sleep because I kept having nightmares. This went on for a few days, and I reported in sick. I began to view the world as a place full of dread and fear. The doctor suggested antidepressants and I took them for a short time, but found that talking about the situation helped far more.

My place of work was helpful in as far as not taking issue with my sickness, but I had little structured support or any form of post-incident debriefing. I made a proactive decision to leave the facility and follow a career path that would lead me to helping those who had experienced similar situations. That has helped me to come to terms with my own experience and regain my perspective on the event.

Case Study Two

I am a sign language interpreter. The incident involved a deaf man who had already had a few outbursts and was being closely observed. He picked up a table and threw it against the window. Other patients scattered, the alarm sounded and several staff were summoned (two from a hearing unit). Three staff grabbed him from behind and two from the front and pulled his legs out from under him. He was very well supported and deftly brought to the ground. When he was down, face down on the floor, he kept his forehead pressed to the floor and kept shouting. I lay down on the floor next to him and tried to get him to look at me. I was told not to touch him, but there was no other way of getting his attention. He eventually calmed down and took notice of what the nurse was saying to him, via my interpretation. He was unable to respond as his arms and hands were held. I remember thinking at the time that the image was one of a rampaging wild animal being captured. Not pleasant. But there was no communication. Staff were speaking to each other and to him and it seemed incredible that they didn't realise he could hear nothing. I can still remember it clearly even though it happened a few years ago. I was quite upset but didn't speak to anyone about it because of the confidentiality issue.

Case Study Three

I have worked with both deaf and hearing people. In the natural course of my work, I hear many life stories that involve physical and sexual abuse. This doesn't usually disturb me or if it does I chat it over with colleagues and I am fine. However, I saw a deaf lady who used a lot of mime in her sign language. Her signing was often very large and her communication very direct. She was not subtle. She told me about her abuse, which I think in anybody's eyes would have been seen as horrific. But there was something so visual about it that it was impossible to get it out of my head later on. I didn't just 'hear' her story, I 'lived' her story as she told it. The pity of it was so huge, made bigger by a large grown-up miming being a small child being beaten, that it seemed to take up my whole visual field so that I could see nothing but the abuse and no longer maintain my role as objective therapist. This lady exhibited challenging behaviours of her own and subsequently I think it was sometimes difficult to untangle thoughts about her dangerousness from the images of her acting out the violence done to her.

Case Study Four

When I was training, I went on a course about PTSD. We split into small groups and were each given a real-life case study to discuss. Our case study was so disgusting, about a woman horribly raped, degraded and assaulted, that I virtually remember it word for word. And that was ten years ago. It was horrible. I wondered about the motivation of the people teaching us. Did they think, 'We have to listen to this all day, so I don't see why you lot shouldn't' or were they so desensitised that they didn't even know that we would be traumatised by it? Honestly, I feel sick when I think about it, even now.

Case Study Five

I used to work for an interpreting agency. A Deaf client in a mental health setting barricaded one of the interpreters I supervised into a room. A social worker and specialist mental health advocate, with whom the client was angry, were also present. The interpreter was not directly threatened at any point but felt threatened by the potential danger of the situation. Eventually, the interpreter made out they needed the toilet, was allowed to leave and then alerted other staff to deal with the situation.

The worst part of all this was the way it was dealt with afterwards. I met the social worker and discussed the situation and found their attitude frustrating. I wanted to make sure interpreters were protected in future. I discussed seating arrangements with them and panic buttons and so on. It felt like the social worker had not considered any potential danger or prevention strategies and certainly had no thought for how the interpreter had felt. They said that in the barricade situation the interpreter had acted professionally and that 'all was fine'. But this was a very different story from what the interpreter told me! I felt like they thought I was overreacting. I had to be really assertive to make my point heard.

HOW DO TRAUMA AND VT AFFECT THE DYNAMICS OF MANAGING CHALLENGING BEHAVIOUR?

It has been suggested that repeated exposure to violence has a greater psychological impact upon those managing challenging behaviour (Wildgoose *et al.*, 2003). The natural symptoms of stress have the potential to influence the practice of such MHPs during similar, future events. It is important to consider the implications of this for practitioners working with such behaviours.

The management dynamics of challenging behaviour are informed by two variables: prediction and prevention, as well as the intervention itself (National Institute for Clinical Excellence (NICE), 2005a).

PREDICTION

The art of prediction arises from the assessment and management of risk. Accurate collection and collation of risk data are important facets of this process, requiring levels of interpersonal skill and data interpretation that will be difficult without the ability to concentrate and think logically. In an MHP who is suffering with trauma or VT, this will be compromised by the symptoms of anxiety, poor sleep and fatigue (Collins and Long, 2003).

Acquiring quality information that will help to design a risk-management care plan will ultimately require information supplied by the service user. A service user's insight into their own behaviour is invaluable in the prediction of violence and aggression and, more importantly, how they usually manage it (NICE, 2005a). If the service user is connected with the MHP's exposure to trauma or VT, the MHP may choose to use avoidance tactics to cope, and therefore miss such vital information. This could take the form of asking others to undertake the assessment or passing on keyworker responsibilities to another. These measures are invariably short term and are unlikely to alleviate the MHP's distress since they will still have to maintain their 'professional shape' while interacting with the service user on the unit.

PREVENTION

In terms of preventive measures, such as the application of de-escalation strategies, the influence of emotional variables upon an emotion-fuelled dynamic become obvious. De-escalation, or diffusing, is a key feature in the prevention of the development of anger into aggression and potential violence (Paterson *et al.*, 1998; Jeffery and Austen, 2005). Intrinsic to de-escalation is the level of self-awareness exhibited by the MHP. This allows the MHP to understand and counter their contribution to the dynamic. How we act and what we say will determine whether anger is perpetuated or resolved.

It has been noted that higher rates of poor professional judgement are more likely in stressed MHPs (Munroe *et al.*, 1995; Stamm, 1997). Anger, irritability and anxiety are factors that are consistent in both managing challenging behaviour and in trauma and VT (Baker and Allen, 2001; Sequeira and Halstead, 2004).

As noted in case study one: the healthcare professional began to view the world as a hostile place and felt that 'the world was a place full of fear and dread'. This is in keeping with the findings of Sequeira and Halstead (2004), who note that increases in anxiety and subsequent irritability can increase the likelihood of staff feeling they have to intervene to minimise the risk to their own safety. The paradox here is that, through hypervigilance, the staff member reacts to their own emotional behaviour rather than that of the service user. It is important to note that anger is the unifying principle in the service user and the staff member during this dynamic. Whittington and Wykes (1994) report that prior confrontations with staff are a factor in perpetuating assaultive behaviour towards specific individuals. The feelings of care staff towards violence and aggression are a factor in their responses to future behaviours by the same service user (Farrell, 1997; Watts and Morgan, 1994).

It is here that avoidance strategies severely impact upon a preventive measure such as de-escalation. Such strategies are dependent upon active engagement and proactive intervention in order to identify escalatory factors while the service user still has better control and reasoning. If staff members avoid key warning signs, the result is reactive rather than proactive practice, since anger will escalate if it continues unchecked, unidentified and unchannelled (Jeffery and Austen, 2005). In sign language environments, where service users are expert readers of body language, the subtle signs of a staff member's trauma, such as jumpiness, tensed body, rapid eye movement and anxious or irritable communication will be picked up more accurately than the equivalent hearing service user. In such situations, subsequent attempts to de-escalate may in fact fuel the aggressive reaction.

Another facet of prevention is that of observation. In this context, observation may be defined as working one to one with an individual with the intention of assessing, monitoring and delivering therapeutic intervention. It is a process that is predominantly undertaken by mental health nurses (Bouic, 2005). But, as Mackay *et al.* (2005) note, the process of observation often fails to recognise the 'abuse or hostility and the potential stress this may cause to the "observing nurse" in close proximity' (p. 465).

This clearly has implications for MHPs who are already emotionally fragile. Effective therapy is based upon a therapist's attentiveness and their timely detection of warning signs, both of which can be affected by their emotional state, which might possibly impede the therapeutic engagement. Blunted affect will ultimately impede an activity that requires emotional control to maintain its therapeutic remit.

INTERVENTION

Physical intervention strategies are a source of moral dilemma for the MHP. Some studies have identified that the memory of holding onto a service user can leave such a lasting impression that a future episode can evoke these memories (Hawkins *et al.*, 2005). This is compounded by their potential contribution to the 'reawakening' of a service user's past experiences of abuse (Smith, 1995; Bonner *et al.*, 2002).

Marangos-Frost and Wells (2000) report a far more alarming variable: that some service users in their study reported that they 'sensed' staff's anger towards them by the way they were held. Emotional response from care staff has been established as a clear risk indicator in the inappropriate use of physical intervention (Hinsby and Baker, 2004). Given the overactive sense of danger and a propensity to emotionally overreact, the MHP with symptoms of VT may not be best placed to remain objective during the assessment of an evolving crisis event.

Sequeira and Halstead (2004) identify factors concerning the psychological effects upon staff using physical interventions within the forensic environment. This work needs to be replicated within deaf services to ascertain parity in results. Collecting the subjective experiences of deaf service users and deaf staff who have been restrained or have restrained others, or have witnessed members of their community being restrained, is of great importance if we are to learn how to minimise the impact of VT.

RECOMMENDATIONS FOR SELF-CARE

It is ethically and professionally important that we ensure that MHPs are aware of the potential occupational hazards inherent in their work.

Self-care is vital when working with service users with challenging behaviour and trauma. It is important in training and qualified work that these issues are discussed and individuals are given the chance to explore their coping strategies.

The following encompass the intrinsic components required of the individual and their employer in order for staff to self-care within the context of trauma and VT:

- **personal therapy**
- **regular supervision**
- **peer support**
- **balance between work, rest and play**
- **balanced caseload**
- **clear boundaries**
- **cultural shift**
- **developments in service provision.**

PERSONAL THERAPY

This helps the MHP to identify and work through issues within their own history. It aims to focus upon unresolved feelings and emergent themes that may impact upon interactions with service users. For deaf members of staff, this may be difficult to achieve due to the scarcity of therapists that can sign. It is likely that a deaf staff member will be well known, in a social or work capacity, to any therapists within sensible commuting distance. This leaves them only with the choice of travelling remarkable distances or to seeing a hearing therapist with an interpreter, which has its own difficulties (Napier and Cornes, 2004).

REGULAR SUPERVISION

Supervision is important in ensuring that the MHP does not become enmeshed in the issues of frequent interaction and intervention. The MHP needs to be aware that they may be vulnerable to the experiences and pain of the service user and remain in touch with their own sense of self. For deaf members of staff, supervision needs to give space to discussing 'small community' issues, e.g. boundary issues of knowing a service user socially and empathy issues when deaf staff and service users share similar life experiences. Sign language interpreters often struggle with issues of appropriate supervision as they tend to be employed on a freelance basis and their occasional employer, despite possibly being best placed and best qualified to do so, takes no responsibility in providing supervision or training on trauma and mental health issues. Napier and Cornes (2004) suggest that the personal experiences of the interpreter will directly influence their reception and production during their work. Impartiality is a requirement of professional interpreters and, without space to explore their own reactions to the traumatic material to which they are exposed, is likely to be jeopardised by the lack of appropriate supervision.

PEER SUPPORT

Working with trauma presents its own potential stressors, and the MHP may often feel isolated. Peer support is often sought by staff in areas where a viable support structure is absent (Jenkins and Elliot, 2004), though there is evidence that many MHPs value the peer support process above any formalised system (Dallender *et al.*, 1999). The important factor here is that a sense of isolation has potential to compound VT; so any opportunity for consistent support is important. Unfortunately, owing to the relatively small number of deaf people employed in mental health services, it may be that deaf staff do not have an obvious peer group with which to discuss issues specific to being deaf in potentially traumatic environments. It is crucial that the opportunity is found for deaf members of staff to meet with staff members from similar services elsewhere, or that hearing and deaf professionals are aware of their potential similarities and differences in their experience of trauma.

For staff working in teams, it is usually made clear to patients that confidentiality is shared within the team rather than with an individual MHP, thus allowing shared debriefs and peer support between team members. The sign language interpreter has a particular difficulty if employed on a freelance basis and working alone as they may find that the rules of confidentiality prevent them discussing their experiences in any detail with anyone else, leaving them isolated and unsupported.

BALANCE BETWEEN WORK, REST AND PLAY

As we become immersed in the world of another, it is all too easy to be consumed by the act of caring. Being able to take time out and engage in the personal pursuits that make us who we are is vital in maintaining our sense of self.

BALANCED CASELOAD

Having exposure to balanced caseloads with service users who have a diverse range of issues can have a significant influence in minimising the impact of VT. For example, McCann and Pearlman (1990) point out that there is a discrete difference between working with trauma survivors and other types of trauma, since the latter exposes the MHP to shocking imagery.

CLEAR BOUNDARIES

Given that deaf staff may know their deaf service users personally from some other walk of life, it is hypothesised that this, along with the increased empathy that Deaf people are likely to share, combines to increase the chances of deaf staff getting VT. The sign language interpreter may also know the service user from previous interpreting jobs and know other traumatic details or information that relate to current trauma. However, owing to ethical constraints, the interpreter may not be able to share this information with their current workplace. This places additional emotional strain on the interpreter and puts them in the situation of having to make ongoing risk assessments as to whether the information they hold affects the safety of the service user or staff, and whether this warrants them breaching previous confidentiality. Without the appropriate training and supervision from MHPs, it is unlikely that the interpreter is best placed to make such risk assessments, and such blurred boundaries could jeopardise patient and staff safety.

The importance of boundaries in the MHP's personal and professional life, the need for debriefing and ongoing professional development and supervision are fundamental factors when working with trauma. Meiselman (1990) identifies a number of warning signals in terms of burnout; these include obsessing about the service user, withdrawing from others and the blurring of therapeutic boundaries.

CULTURAL SHIFT

It would also be important to introduce a culture whereby acknowledging the impact of the work is a strength rather than a weakness. An important facet of coping with the intensity of the work is to acknowledge it will affect you and that it's OK to feel shocked, saddened or vulnerable.

DEVELOPMENTS IN SERVICE PROVISION

In the course of selecting and training MHPs, more emphasis should perhaps be placed on the realities of the job in terms of the demands in today's NHS. One might argue that a core part of the MHP's curriculum should be devoted to personal stress management and coping skills.

The literature clearly identifies that through the use of these strategies professionals can reduce the likelihood of not only trauma and VT but also the effects of burnout (NICE, 2005b). In addition, we need to ensure that trainee MHPs are prepared for the impact of working with service users and are able to meet the inherent challenges.

CONCLUSION

It has been suggested that those exposed to traumatic events are likely to exhibit symptoms of PTSD within a week (NICE, 2005b). What has not been explored, however, is that MHPs working with ongoing challenging behaviour and trauma may not have the opportunity to 'recover'. There is a clear need for further study in this area as it can be reasoned that this may have consequences for both the prediction and prevention of violence. It will most likely influence and guide the decision-making process in terms of the use of interventions. Staff behaviour will ultimately be guided by their experiences of previous events and as such these may contribute to both the escalation of anger and the interactions during the crisis event.

There is a need for increased awareness and training as to the impact of working with service users who exhibit challenging behaviour and those who are traumatised, and its impact on the MHP. The literature is clear that individuals who work with service users who have experienced trauma need ongoing support. Conversely, the literature also predicts that personal, professional and organisational support may provide protective factors to mediate against some of the risks relating to the development of trauma and VT. Furthermore, it is essential that supervision is part of the individual's working life, promoting both their personal and professional development. Most of all, a culture that supports and values staff and promotes their care should be cultivated in supporting staff in working with challenging behaviour. However, such support and supervision may be difficult for deaf staff and sign language interpreters to access, when compared to hearing staff.

An understanding and awareness of countertransference and empathy is crucial in our work and is particularly important for deaf staff and children of deaf adults who work with deaf service users. The greater impact of receiving information in the more visual sign language on VT needs further research. It is imperative that individuals are made more aware of the psychological impact of working with service users and the impact this work might potentially have on the MHP's sense of self and identity. The lack of insight by MHPs into this phenomenon may have a huge impact on their own emotional and psychological health.

Discourse with deaf people in the context of both trauma and VT is currently an area of neglect and needs to given greater priority in the future.

REFERENCES

Allen JG (1995) *Coping with Trauma: A Guide to Self-Understanding*, Washington, American Psychiatric Press.

American Psychiatric Association (2000) *Diagnostic and Statistical Manual of Mental Disorders* (4th edn.), Washington, American Psychiatric Association.

Baker P, Allen D (2001) Physical abuse and physical interventions in learning disabilities: an element of risk? *Journal of Adult Protection* 3(2): 25–31.

Barker P (2002) The tidal model: the healing potential of metaphor within the patient's narrative. *Journal of Psychosocial Nursing* 40(7): 43–50.

Barker P, Buchanan-Barker P (2004) Beyond empowerment: revering the story-teller. *Mental Health Practice* 7(5): 18–20.

Bloom SL, Reichert M (1998) *Bearing Witness: Violence and Collective Responsibility*, New York, The Haworth Press.

Bonner G, Lowe T, Rawcliffe D, Wellman N (2002) Trauma for all: a pilot study of the subjective experience of physical restraint for mental health in-patients and staff in the UK. *Journal of Psychiatric and Mental Health Nursing* 9(4): 465–73.

Bouic L (2005) Focus on psychiatric observation. *Mental Health Practice* 8(8): 17–19.

British Deaf Association (1999) *Sign Language Policy*, London, British Deaf Association.

Collins S, Long A (2003) Too tired to care? The psychological effects of working with trauma. *Journal of Psychiatric and Mental Health Nursing* 10(1): 17–27.

Dallender J, Nolan P, Soares J, Thomsen S, Arnetz B (1999) A comparative study of the perceptions of British mental health nurses and psychiatrists of their work environment. *Journal of Advanced Nursing* 29(1): 36–43.

Farrell GA (1997) Aggression in clinical settings: nurses' views. Journal of Advanced Nursing 25(3): 501–8.

Figley CR (1995) *Compassion Fatigue*, New York, Brunner Mazel.

Friedman MJ (1997) Posttraumatic stress disorder. *Journal of Clinical Psychiatry* 58(suppl 9): 33–6.

Freud A (1959) *The Ego and the Mechanisms of Defence*, London, Karnac.

Harvey MA (2001) Vicarious emotional trauma of interpreters: a clinical psychologist's perspective. *Journal of Interpretation* 1: 85–98.

Hawkins S, Allen D, Jenkins R (2005) The use of physical interventions with people with intellectual disabilities and challenging behaviour: the experiences of service users and staff members. *Journal of Applied Research in Intellectual Disabilities* 18(1): 19–34.

Healthcare Commission (2005) *The National Audit of Violence (2003–2005): Final Report*, London, Royal College of Psychiatrists Research Unit.

Herman JL (1992) *Trauma and Recovery: The Aftermath of Violence*, New York, Basic Books.

Herman JL (1997) *Trauma and Recovery: The Aftermath of Violence from Domestic Violence Abuse to Political Terror*, New York, Basic Books.

Hinsby K, Baker M (2004) Patient and nurse accounts of violent incidents in a medium secure unit. *Journal of Psychiatric and Mental Health Nursing* 11(3): 341–7.

Horowitz MJ (1986) *Stress Response Syndromes*, Northvale, NJ, Jason Aronson.

Jeffery D, Austen S (2005) Adapting de-escalation techniques with deaf service users. *Nursing Standard* 19(49): 41–7.

Jenkins R, Elliot P (2004) Stressors, burnout and social support: nurses in acute mental health settings. *Journal of Advanced Nursing* 48(6): 622–31.

Mackay I, Paterson B, Cassells C (2005) Constant or special observations of inpatients presenting a risk of aggression or violence: nurses' perceptions of the rules of engagement. *Journal of Psychiatric and Mental Health Nursing* 12(4): 464–71.

Marangos-Frost S, Wells D (2000) Psychiatric nurses' thoughts and feelings about restraint use: a decision dilemma. *Journal of Advanced Nursing* 31(2): 362–9.

McCann IL, Pearlman LA (1990) Vicarious traumatisation: a framework for understanding the psychological effects of working with victims. *Journal of Traumatic Stress* 3(1): 131–49.

McCay V, Andrews JF (1990) *The Psychology of Deafness: Understanding Deaf and Hard of Hearing People*, New York, Longman.

McSwain K, Robinson R, Pantelu L (1998) Vicarious Trauma: Bearing Witness to Another's Trauma, http://www.drjontry.com/handouts/vicarious.htm, accessed 1 February 2005.

Meiselman KC (1990) *Resolving the Trauma of Incest: Reintegration Therapy with Survivors*, San Francisco, Jossey-Bass.

Merriam-Webster (2003) *Merriam-Webster's Collegiate Dictionary* (11th edn.), Springfield, MA, Encyclopaedia Britannica Publishing Company.

Munroe JF, Shay J, Fisher L, Makary C *et al.* (1995) Preventing compassion fatigue: a team treatment model. In Figley CR (ed), *Compassion Fatigue: Coping with Secondary Traumatic Stress in Those who Treat the Traumatized*, Bristol, PA, Brunner Mazel, pp. 209–32.

Napier J, Cornes A (2004) The dynamic role of interpreters and therapists. In Austen S, Crocker S (eds), *Deafness in Mind: Working Psychologically with Deaf People Across the Lifespan*, London, Whurr, pp. 161–79.

National Audit Office (2003) *A Safer Place to Work: Protecting NHS Hospital and Ambulance Staff from Violence and Aggression*, London, TSO.

National Institute for Clinical Excellence (2005a) *The Short-term Management of Disturbed/Violent Behaviour in In-patient Psychiatric Settings and Emergency Departments*, London, TSO.

National Institute for Clinical Excellence (2005b) *Post Traumatic Stress Disorder (PTSD): the Management of PTSD in Adults and Children in Primary and Secondary Care: Clinical Guideline 26*, London, NICE.

Paterson B, Leadbetter D, McComish A (1998) De-escalation in the management of aggression and violence. *Nursing Times* 93(36): 58–61.

Pearlman LA, MacIan PS (1995) Vicarious traumatisations: An empirical study of the effects of trauma work on trauma therapists. *Professional Psychology: Research and Practice* 26: 558–65.

Pearlman LA, Saakvitne KW (1995) *Trauma and the Therapist: Counter-Transference and Vicarious Traumatisation in Psychotherapy with Incest Survivors*, New York, WW Norton.

Royal National Institute for Deaf People (1998) *Breaking the Sound Barrier*, London, Royal National Institute for Deaf People.

Sequeira H, Halstead S (2004) The psychological effects on nursing staff of administering physical restraint in a secure psychiatric hospital: 'When I go home, it's then that I think about it.' *British Journal of Forensic Practice* 6(1): 3–15.

Smith SB (1995) Restraints: retraumatization for rape victims? *Journal of Psychosocial Nursing and Mental Health Services* 33(7): 23–28.

Stamm H (1997) Work-related secondary traumatic stress. *PTSD Research Quarterly* 8(2): 25–34.

Sullivan P, Brookhauser P, Scanlan M (2000) Maltreatment of deaf and hard of hearing children. In Hindley P, Kitson N (eds), *Mental Health and Deafness*, London, Whurr, pp. 149–84.

Watts D, Morgan G (1994) Malignant alienation: dangers for patients who are hard to like. *British Journal of Psychiatry* 164(5): 11–15.

Whittington R, Wykes T (1994) Going in strong: confrontative coping by staff following assault by a patient. *Journal of Forensic Psychiatry* 5: 609–14.

Wildgoose J, Briscoe M, Lloyd K (2003) Psychological and emotional problems in staff following assaults by patients. *Psychiatric Bulletin* 27(8): 697–8.

4

Diagnosis and Challenging Behaviour of Deaf People

SALLY AUSTEN, ALISON GRAY AND STEVE CARNEY

INTRODUCTION

This chapter looks at the purpose, effectiveness and integrity of diagnosis and its applicability to deaf people with challenging behaviour. Anger is a normal feature of Western society, although aggression is usually seen as problematic. In this chapter, the aetiology of aggression in relation to mental ill health and learning disability is discussed. Rates of misdiagnosis in deaf people are extremely high and affect both treatment and human rights. Paucity of research evidence, communication problems on the part of the client and the clinician and the complexity of dual and multiple diagnoses compound the difficulties of diagnosis in deaf people.

WHAT IS CHALLENGING BEHAVIOUR?

Emerson (1995) defines challenging behaviour as: 'culturally abnormal behaviour(s) of such an intensity, frequency or duration that the physical safety of the person or others is likely to be placed in serious jeopardy, or behaviour which is likely to seriously limit use of, or result in, the person being denied access to ordinary community facilities' (p. 44). This covers a broad spectrum of behaviour, including self-injury, violence towards others and damage to property. What is defined

Deafness and Challenging Behaviour: The 360° Perspective. Edited by S. Austen and D. Jeffery
© 2007 John Wiley & Sons Ltd

as challenging will vary between settings and with the capacity of others (family, staff, authorities) to manage difficult behaviour.

The norms and expectations of society determine which behaviours are acceptable and which are deemed challenging. This fluctuates over time and the specific situation. For example, expressing physical aggression as a soldier in wartime will be positively rewarded; expressing the same aggression back home on leave leads to problems.

WHAT IS DIAGNOSIS?

Diagnosis refers to the identification of diseases from the examination of symptoms. To identify symptoms, an analysis of the individual's unique condition, their social situation and their environment is required. Thus, challenging behaviour should be analysed at different levels:

- the individual
- the local (the immediate environment)
- the social (the norms and expectations of society).

A diagnosis is a clinical label that allows practitioners to group people who have similar problems together. Without such diagnostic categories, the clinician would not be able to compare past or present cases to identify the best treatment. Diagnosis is a fine art, and behaviours that appear similar may in fact have very different causes. Accurate diagnosis enables clinicians to undertake research and learn from other people's experiences. Diagnosis allows for prediction of the likely course of any illness and identifies the most appropriate treatment. International classifications of disease such as the World Health Organization's *International Statistical Classification of Diseases and Related Health Problems, Tenth Revision* (ICD-10) (WHO, 1992) and the *Diagnostic and Statistical Manual of Mental Disorders* (DSM-IV) (American Psychiatric Association, 1994) enable clinicians to communicate opinions about diagnosis clearly across international boundaries.

DIFFICULTIES IN THE DIAGNOSIS OF DEAF PEOPLE

Deaf people are prone to under- and over-diagnosis (Denmark, 1985). Over-diagnosis impacts on the human rights of the individual, and under-diagnosis results in patients being neglected. Shapira *et al.* (1999) found that 70.8% of deaf patients with bipolar disorder and 56.7% of other deaf patients had an inaccurate discharge diagnosis, which did not improve on multiple admissions.

A greater understanding of deafness, Deaf culture, sign language in hearing professionals and an increase in the number of deaf professionals is necessary to improve this situation. However, it is not only hearing people that have negative assumptions about deaf patients. Dickert (1988) found that, while staff in specialist deaf provision had generally more positive attitudes, deaf and hearing staff were more likely to describe deaf patients as needing supervision and medication than equivalent hearing patients. Within specialist services, some professionals have never met healthy deaf sign language users and attribute as common to deaf people that which is only common to deaf people with additional disabilities.

DIAGNOSIS AS A TOOL OF SOCIAL POWER

Diagnoses provide useful categorisation but can be misused as tools of social power. Lane (1993) says that mental health clinicians have real power over deaf people but often function on knowledge gleaned from hearing stereotypes, such as 'deafness equates to stupidity'. He describes the contradictory findings of prevalence studies and remarks that 'Such diagnostic mayhem not only leads to irresponsible characterizations of deaf people; it prevents effective planning of the services deaf people need' (p. 55). Lane suggests that research methodology is also affected by the hearing clinician's stereotypes and refutes prevalence studies that say that deaf people have higher rates of challenging behaviour than hearing people. Griggs (2004) suggests that 'traditionally mental health professionals have used normative criteria to define mental health and illness, and in doing so have seen normality and deviance through the cultural lens of the dominant group in society' (p. 115). She recommends the Wellness Model, in which a 'pathology' framework is replaced by an exploration of what goes right in the psychological development and adjustment of the individual, for working with deaf sign language users.

RESEARCH AND DIAGNOSIS

Accurate diagnosis depends on access to international evidence-based literature and research. Data are relatively sparse in the field of mental health and deafness, both nationally and internationally. This is due to a number of reasons.

- There are relatively few professionals working in mental health and deafness, most of whom have to prioritise the shorter-term clinical needs of their patients over longer-term research needs. There are very few deaf professionals.
- Few measures, tests or questionnaires have been validated for use with deaf people and even fewer for sign language users.
- Measures can lose validity and reliability when translated into sign language or are invalidated by being presented in written form, as the average reading age of the deaf adult is below literate levels (Mayberry, 2002).
- There is no register of deaf people in the UK, and often the means of identifying them (e.g. through social services) excludes the highest functioning and skews the population. Likewise, some of the lowest functioning people will be excluded as they may be in institutions and/or not identified by their audiological status so much as their additional needs.
- Deaf people are not a homogeneous group owing to the huge variations in cause and degree of deafness and experiences associated with deafness. Research sample sizes are often too small to be significant.
- Research areas that are little understood, such as deafness, attract little funding, which means they remain little understood.

LANGUAGE, COMMUNICATION AND SKILLS OF THE SERVICE USER

Language and communication skills are crucial to diagnostic interview. However, many people who are born deaf experience severely delayed and impoverished language skills regardless of mode of expression (whether it be spoken language or sign language) (Mayberry, 2002). An example is that in a study by Gregory *et al.* (1995) nearly 20% of the deaf school leavers interviewed were not able to complete an interview in either sign language or speech despite all being of normal IQ.

Once an individual has language delay, the language and communication problems not only influence the progress of the diagnostic interview but can also inhibit differential diagnosis by mimicking other symptoms. For example, language deprivation and incomplete development of the Theory of Mind (the ability to think that other's think differently to us) can result in someone of normal IQ functioning in society as if they had a global learning disability.

Diagnosis requires the greatest possible degree of shared language in order for the patient to describe their often complex and confusing internal experiences to the clinician. Often even with deaf staff and perfect interpretation this is not directly possible for those deaf people who have reduced language. In this situation, diagnosis depends on collecting as much information as possible from the patient and carers and then testing out a trial treatment or intervention. In many cases, an accurate diagnosis is only possible with an admission to a specialist deaf mental health service employing staff with whom the patient can communicate fully. It can also assist diagnosis to observe interaction with other deaf patients in this setting.

Denmark (1966), having worked with deaf people with mental health problems, suggests that anger can escalate into aggression when deaf people have difficulty expressing themselves: 'the inability to express dissatisfaction or anger by emotionally toned verbalizations often leads to the physical display of such feelings. These reactions, at times explosive in nature, are incomprehensible and may be mistaken for the manifestations of mental illness' (p. 121). (It is language rather than specifically audition that is required for self-expression: either words or signs are sufficient (Mayberry, 2002).) However, regardless of language competence, deaf people will often be misunderstood by hearing people. This may increase the frustration of a deaf person and, as Denmark (1966) says, increase the chance of misdiagnosis. O'Rourke and Beail (2004) believe that deaf people are more suggestible than hearing people due to a paucity of experience and information, heightened anxiety and being less assertive in interviews with hearing professionals. This could result in them being inappropriately charged with crimes or diagnosed with mental illness. They also report that the nature of British Sign Language, where examples of sample answers are often given to support a question, plays a part in suggestibility.

Gray and du Feu (2004) report that communication difficulties can make diagnosis of the deaf service user particularly difficult as subtle changes in behaviour in the early stages of illness may be missed. Hearing families may not sign enough to detect such changes.

LANGUAGE, COMMUNICATION AND SKILLS OF THE CLINICIAN

Gray and du Feu (2004) highlight the fact that, although the first point of assessment for mental health problems in the UK is usually primary care, the tendency for GPs to lack Deaf awareness results in deaf patients avoiding them. They suggest that 'greater investment in Deaf awareness training, communication technologies and in interpreter training to bring equity of access to Deaf patients is required to maximize the chance of accurate and timely diagnosis' (p. 209). Deaf people rarely have interpreter assistance in GP surgeries and often rely on family support, even for matters of a very personal and intimate nature (Reeves *et al.*, 2003). Thacker (1991) cautions that professionals who try to communicate with deaf clients by writing can mistake poor literacy for disordered thinking.

Kitson and Thacker (2000) suggest that non-specialist mental health workers will be less able to elicit facts or observe communication and that incorrect treatment and prolonged hospitalisation can result. It is therefore crucial that clinicians are as versed as possible in the culture and language of their patients. The assessment of deaf people on a general (hearing) psychiatric ward is difficult because of the lack of signing staff, the scarcity of interpreters with mental health experience and the lack of funding for regular interpreter use. Even with interpreters, non-specialist staff may struggle. Harry (1986) cautions that interviews conducted through a sign language interpreter may inhibit the interaction and therefore diagnosis. Without knowledge of the norms of sign language, some features may be mistaken for pathological symptoms. For example, repeating a sign to ensure it is understood may be diagnosed as perseveration, and rapid topic changes and talking past the point (a defence against poor comprehension) may be mistaken for thought disorder. Even fluent signers can assume the signs of others are representative of disorder if there are strong regional, dialectical or age differences in the patient's sign (Thacker, 1994; Thacker, 2001).

Where there is a need for compulsory detainment under the Mental Health Act 1983, there is a statutory requirement for approved social workers to take into account any hearing or linguistic difficulties the patient may have and to interview patients in a 'suitable manner'. There is not, however, the same requirement of doctors (Hindley, *et al.*, 2000). Hindley *et al.* were so concerned by misdiagnosis by non-deaf specialists that they recommended that all deaf patients detained under any mental health law should have their detention and treatment reviewed by a specialist psychiatrist of deaf people.

Hindley *et al.* (1993) found that the outcome of psychiatric assessments of signing deaf children and adolescents was affected by the interviewer's signing ability and cultural status. Poor linguistic competence on the part of the interviewer resulted in a reduction in the range of symptoms elicited at interview and a masking of a child's emotional difficulties. Sometimes, the deaf client has such an ability with language that they can 'code-switch' (assess the language needs of the clinician and move to a different form of communication accordingly). In reality, this usually means moving away from British Sign Language, with its own unique grammar structure, to Sign Supported English or even mime and speech. Lane (1993) cautions that in these cases the service user is seen to have had social empathy and insight and the clinician may conclude that 'the deaf person must be mentally healthy. If, on the other hand, the psychiatrist cannot communicate fluently with the deaf person, then the deaf person is no doubt ill' (p, 54).

ANGER, BEHAVIOUR DISORDER AND CHALLENGING BEHAVIOUR

Behavioural problems are reported to be more prevalent in the deaf population than in the hearing community (Schlesinger and Meadow, 1972; Freeman *et al.*, 1981; Hindley, 2000). Challenging behaviour in deaf people may be an expression of anger or frustration or may indicate a mental health problem or learning disability.

Anger is a normal human emotion and one that arguably deaf people, who are disproportionately disadvantaged and discriminated against (RNID, 1998), have more than a right to feel. In the Western world, expressions of anger and frustration are broadly acceptable as long as they steer clear of aggressive or destructive behaviour. The appropriateness of the ways of expressing anger, however, will depend on context. For example, expressing anger by shouting may be socially acceptable during a football match, but not so during a funeral.

A degree of difficult and challenging behaviour is a normal part of childhood development. All children need to test out boundaries and learn what is and is not socially acceptable. Some deaf people may never have learned what behaviour is reasonable. Bond (2000) suggests that inappropriate reinforcement of bad behaviour is often the root of this. He gives the example of children who have life-threatening conditions and who subsequently and consequently receive high levels of attention from their parents regardless of the appropriateness of their behaviour. Bad behaviour escalates if people are shielded from the consequences of their actions. Deaf people often are. Even within the criminal justice system, professionals feel sorry for the deaf person and drop charges. Vernon and Miller (2005) suggest that some prosecutions do not proceed because the investigating officer cannot to be bothered to arrange interpreters and fill in extra paperwork.

Although both DSM-IV and ICD-10 have diagnostic categories for child behavioural disorders, in practice the boundaries between 'normal' behaviour and pathological behaviour are fluid. Depending on how the behavioural problem or disorder is defined Freeman *et al.* (1981) conclude that 7–10% of hearing children and 20–30% of deaf children are affected.

MENTAL HEALTH PROBLEMS AND CHALLENGING BEHAVIOUR

The link between mental health problems and challenging behaviour can be coincidental or causal. It has not yet been established whether deaf people experience mental illnesses with the same incidence as hearing people, but there are arguments to suggest that some illnesses, such as schizophrenia, may be more prevalent in the deaf people due to social exclusion and life stresses, lack of access to adequate treatment and poor coping mechanisms (Gray and du Feu, 2004).

PSYCHOSIS

Psychosis can be caused by drug misuse and physical illness but most commonly by mental illness, such as schizophrenia. A psychotic illness is one in which the individual is cut off from reality and may experience hallucinations and delusions. Atkinson (2006) reports that deaf people experience auditory hallucinations in different ways depending on their degree and onset of hearing loss. Psychotic behaviour may be unpredictable, bizarre and violent. Media coverage has encouraged a rather clichéd image of people with mental illness as dangerous. While people suffering psychotic illnesses, such as schizophrenia, do occasionally commit acts of extreme violence, in reality most people with these illnesses are no more violent than average, even when acutely ill. People with psychotic illnesses are much more likely to harm themselves or be victims of violence than harm other people (Read and Baker, 1996). Aggressive behaviour may be triggered in those with a psychotic mental illness by command hallucinations, experienced by hearing people as the voices ordering them to do things. A study carried out on hearing patients in an acute psychiatric unit concluded that 13.7% of patients admitted were classified as aggressive. Most of these patients suffered from schizophrenia or bipolar affective disorder. However, most aggression was associated with a small number of patients (6%) (Barlow *et al.*, 2000).

Misdiagnosis of psychosis in deaf people has been reported by Denmark (1966) and Kitson and Thacker (2000). Kitson and Fry (1990) note that normal mumbling in sign can be misinterpreted as hallucinosis in deaf peple and that apparently abnormal explanations or beliefs may be explained by lack of vicarious learning or naivety. Gray and du Feu (2004) suggest that odd behaviour which is the result of psychosis can often be blamed on the deafness alone. They also suggest that thought disorder is difficult to establish if the individual's communication is limited and normal baseline language functioning is unclear.

Farroq and Fear (2003) found that people express more psychotic content when interviewed in their first language. Gray and du Feu (2004) conclude from this that the use of sign language interpreters with deaf people is likely to give falsely low rates of psychosis.

MOOD DISORDER

While it is uncommon for those suffering from depression to present challenging behaviour, those with agitated depression can experience intense anxiety, restlessness, irritability and anger resulting in outbursts of aggression.

'Mania' describes a variety of symptoms including inappropriate elation, extreme motor activity, impulsiveness and excessively rapid thought and speech. Challenging behaviour such as this may be the first sign of an affective disorder (mood disorder) of a depressive or bipolar (manic-depressive) illness type. For example, wild sexual experimentation in someone of previously reserved character may suggest mania. The mood may be predominantly happy but can be irritable and angry. Untreated mania often leads to seriously irresponsible and risky behaviour. Challenging behaviour in mania may occur particularly when someone is irritable and has poor impulse control.

In established mania, the person's communication is more rapid, pressured and may be difficult to follow. Mania in deaf sign language users people presents similarly to that in the hearing population with rapid signing, and rapid shifts of attention. This puts particular pressure on the non-native signer or on a sign langauge interpreter inexperienced in working in mental health settings.

Shapira *et al.* (1999) are concerned that bipolar disorder in profoundly prelingually deaf patients is frequently underdiagnosed and that an overemphasis on overt behavioural manifestaions of mania may lead to a diagnosis of schizophrenia instead of bipolar disorder in deaf patients. In their study nine out of eleven deaf patients diagnosed with schizophrenia were found to have clear-cut mood disorder.

DRUG AND ALCOHOL MISUSE

Alcohol is strongly linked to challenging behaviour, particularly aggression and violence (Graham *et al.*, 1998). Excessive consumption leads to disinhibition and risk-taking, impaired decision-making, poorer reflexes and aggression. Challenging behaviour can result directly from the use of some drugs. For example, some people who experience paranoid psychotic states as a result of using amphetamines or phencyclidine (angel dust) lash out in fear for their lives. Indirectly, drugs link to challenging behaviour in that users may engage in violent robbery in order to fund their habit. There are few studies on the prevalence of drug and alcohol problems in the Deaf community in the UK. Austen and Checinski (2000) surmise that deaf people have similar levels of addictive behaviour to hearing people but with much less access to information and services. Dye and Kyle (2001) demonstrate higher than recommended levels of alcohol consumption in all deaf groups, particularly women on higher incomes and men aged 18–24. Davidson (2002) investigated alcohol use in deaf psychiatric patients and found a prevalence of alcohol use disorder of 24%, as opposed to 8–15% in hearing mental health service users.

PERSONALITY DISORDERS

People with personality disorders have patterns of relating to and perceiving the environment that are deeply ingrained, maladaptive and cause impairment in social and behavioural functioning. Various diagnostic subdivisions and conditions are characterised by combinations of anxiety, rigidity, poor impulse-control, immaturity, enhanced aggression and hostility, need for immediate gratification and substance abuse. Personality disorder tends to start in childhood or adolescence and persist throughout adult life, although there is some waning of symptoms in older age.

Where difficult and antisocial behaviour has been long-standing, the diagnosis of antisocial personality disorder (previously known as psychopathic or sociopathic personality disorder) may be used. Persons with this personality disorder callously disregard the rights and feelings of others and exploit others for materialistic gain and personal gratification. Hostility and serious violence is common and they show no remorse for their behaviour. People with these tendencies may commit serious sexual and violent crimes. There is no research currently available on the prevalence of antisocial personality disorder in deaf people, although it is likely to be the same or higher than in hearing people. This diagnosis is likely to be complicated by the restricted development of the Theory of Mind in deaf children of hearing parents and by impairments in understanding the motivation and actions of other people and in moral reasoning that can result from impoverished early education and language deprivation.

Paranoid personality disorder describes individuals who are not psychotic but who commonly react with suspicion and find hostile and malevolent motives behind other people's innocent, trivial or even positive acts. Merck (2006) comments that paranoid tendencies may develop among persons who feel particularly alienated because of a 'defect or handicap' and gives as an example 'a person with chronic deafness may mistakenly think he is being talked about or laughed at'. Although Deaf or deafened people are as likely as hearing people to develop paranoid personality disorders, it is also important to remember that deaf people genuinely do experience high levels of discrimination and harassment (RNID, 1998); it can be extremely anxiety-provoking to lose one's hearing and not be able to access aural information fully; and negative emotional reactions to the oft-experienced isolation and loneliness of deafness are to be expected.

Historically, deaf people have been diagnosed with personality disorders when their presentation is actually the result of impoverished language and educational experiences. Unfortunately, the outdated concept of a 'surdophrenia' (Basilier, 1964) has been resurrected by Vernon and Miller (2005) and renamed 'primitive personality disorder'. This takes the 'symptoms' of minimal language skills, illiteracy, lack of adequate education, 'pervasive cognitive deprivation' (e.g. inability to follow recipes, plan a budget or understand social security) and a performance IQ of above 70 (i.e. not globally learning disabled) to create a diagnosis of primitive personality disorder. In order to provide additional help, it is useful to identify people who are not globally learning disabled but who have difficulty with activities of daily living. However, it seems entirely inappropriate to categorise this as a personality disorder.

AGE-RELATED DIFFICULTIES

Dementia occurs in 6% of the hearing population aged over 65 years (Lobo *et al.*, 2000), and there is no evidence to show that this is different in deaf people. In hearing older people challenging behaviour is twice as common in those with cognitive impairment as those without (Cohen-Mansfield *et al.*, 1990). There is no such prevalence research in deaf older populations. Given the higher rate of problem behaviours in deaf children, it is likely that this prevalence will persist and that premorbid presentation may complicate later diagnoses. The cause of challenging behaviour in older adults is not restricted to organic brain disorder. Confusion resulting from physical illness, stress, sensory deprivation and overstimulation can all be causes. When not able to stay at home, Deaf older adults are often housed in hearing provision leaving them linguistically isolated, lonely and bored (Austen, 2004). Andrews (2006) discusses difficulties in managing challenging behaviour in hearing people in such settings, especially with regard to reducing the need for environmental restraint and psychotropic medication and increasing psychological and psychosocial interventions. It is also important to recognise the role of staff behaviour in determining that of residents.

LEARNING DISABILITY AND CHALLENGING BEHAVIOUR

In this context, 'learning disability' refers to global developmental delay or intellectual impairment. The prevalence of learning disability in total is 3% of the population (2.5% mild, 0.4% moderate and 0.1% severe/profound) (Roeleveld *et al.*, 1997).

THE DIAGNOSIS OF DEAFNESS IN LEARNING-DISABLED PEOPLE

People with learning disabilities are difficult to test audiologically. Lack of deaf awareness by care staff means that people with learning disabilities rarely arrange for clients to receive either initial or ongoing audiological assessments (Timehin and Timehin, 2004), despite a body of evidence that deafness is associated with certain causes of learning disability, e.g. cytomegalovirus, anoxia, prematurity, Down's syndrome and rubella. Research involving carers' identification of hearing impairment in people with learning disabilities results in underestimates (approximately 10%), whereas audiological assessment shows the prevalence of hearing impairment in this group to be about 40% (Yeates, 1995) and for some specific disorders, such as Down's syndrome, it can be as high as 80–95% (Cunningham, 1982).

PREVALENCE OF CHALLENGING BEHAVIOUR IN LEARNING-DISABLED PEOPLE

The prevalence of challenging behaviour in people with learning disability is between 10% and 15% (Emerson *et al.*, 2001). The prevalence of challenging behaviour in deaf children has been reported as three times higher than in hearing children (Schlesinger and Meadow, 1972). However, the prevalence of challenging behaviour in people who are both deaf and learning-disabled is reported as 62% by Timehin and Timehin (2004). They suggest that this high prevalence needs further research to see whether combined learning disability and hearing impairment amplifies problem behaviours or masks psychiatric disorders. People who have a dual diagnosis of learning disability and mental illness are more likely to display challenging behaviour (Borthwick-Duffy, 1994).

DIAGNOSIS OF LEARNING DISABILITY IN DEAF PEOPLE

The diagnosis of learning disability in deaf people is made challenging for two reasons. First, there are extremely few tests that are normed, validated or reliable for use with deaf people. Most instructions require verbal communication, and many test items discriminate against deaf people (Cromwell, 2005). Secondly, most tests measure academic achievement and, aside from low intelligence, there are many reasons connected with communication and access to education that can impair a deaf person's test performance.

The average IQ of the general population is 100 demonstrated across combined verbal and non-verbal subtests. Verbal subtests are rarely valid for use with deaf people as they tend to reflect the degree of residual hearing of the client and the communication skills and determination of the client's teachers, rather than reflecting the true ability of the deaf person. Braden (1994) reports that the use of only performance subtests to reach a global IQ score for deaf people is valid. Mean non-verbal IQ for deaf children with no additional disability is in the normal range (Braden, 1992). However, additional disabilities bring the IQ scores down significantly (Schildroth, 1976). As many as 40%

of deaf children have additional disabilities (Crocker and Edwards, 2004).

Williams and Austen (2000) discuss a 'hidden population' of hearing-impaired people who were misdiagnosed as learning-disabled and languished in institutions until the movement towards community care in the UK (beginning in the 1980s) when their audiological and communication needs were better met. Since community care, however, it is the authors' observation that misdiagnosis commonly occurs in the other direction: that deaf people's specific and global learning disabilities are not diagnosed and they fend for themselves in the community with insufficient support.

DELAYED LANGUAGE AND SPECIFIC LEARNING DISABILITIES

Depressed and delayed language development in deaf children is common but, as a group, not causally related to general intellectual deficiencies in cognitive domains that function independently of language. However, it can lead to poor reading achievement and, on average, the reading age of deaf people is below literate levels (Mayberry, 2002). It can also lead to significant underdevelopment of Theory of Mind skills (Peterson and Siegal, 1999), which markedly affects the understanding of social interaction, rules, empathy and behavioural expectations.

FUNCTIONAL ANALYSIS VERSUS DIAGNOSIS IN CHALLENGING BEHAVIOUR

Challenging behaviour, rather than being symptomatic of a particular condition or diagnosis, may serve a function. Functional analysis – identifying the specific function of the behaviour and finding more appropriate ways of fulfilling it – is often associated with the field of learning disability. However, it is equally useful with deaf people with mental health problems.

CHALLENGING BEHAVIOUR AS A MEANS OF COMMUNICATION BEHAVIOUR

Communication difficulties have long been linked to challenging behaviour, and more recently an inverse (but not causal) relationship has been noted between communication ability and prevalence of challenging behaviour in people with learning disabilities (Sigafoos, 2000). Challenging behaviour in people with learning disabilities may represent an attempt to communicate a message, such as a need to avoid a stressor or need for attention. Interventions are focused on improving the expressive skills of the client that are functionally equivalent, but more socially acceptable. These presentations are equally likely in deaf people who do not have a formal learning disability but who are struggling to communicate, for whatever reason.

Case Study

Williams and Austen (2000) describe the treatment of a deaf man with mild learning disability diagnosed with psychopathic personality disorder. They hypothesise that the client was so terrified of his own anger (probably having picked up from staff with poor sign that anger was bad, as opposed to aggression being bad) that he controlled himself enormously, withheld every complaint and concern and would occasionally explode with extreme violence when the 'final straw broke the camel's back'. Treatment involved educating this man to use anger as a potentially positive motivator of change. The client was equipped with words and signs to express his emotions, and a numbering system on a scale of 0–10, with ten being out-of-control anger that results in violence. He was able to learn to express and negotiate when mildly angry and to recognise potential danger and leave the situation before getting dangerously angry.

Challenging behaviour can also indicate a lack of receptive comprehension. Kevan (2003) highlights the tendency of staff to overestimate the receptive skill of people with learning disabilities and challenging behaviour, and Yeates (1992) regards unrecognised hearing loss as a cause of challenging behaviour.

CHALLENGING BEHAVIOUR AS A RESULT OF STRESS

Someone who is living with both learning disability and deafness experiences a 'double jeopardy' (Williams and Austen, 2000). Living with a learning disability in 'normal' society often means in reality a lack of employment, which could lead to low self-esteem, a lack of control over their life choices, such as where or with whom they live, and feeling different or trying to 'pass' to fit in with the majority. This is also the case for people who are deaf and have mental health problems. When people are under stress, their tolerance and ability to inhibit fight-or-flight mechanisms are reduced, therefore making challenging behaviour more likely. People who have periods of disturbed sleep are also more prone to challenging behaviour (Kiernan and Kiernan, 1994).

CHALLENGING BEHAVIOUR AND PHYSICAL CONDITIONS

For deaf people, challenging behaviour may occur in the absence of mental illness, for example when struggling to communicate physical distress: toothache may present as headbanging or stomach pain as increased irritability and anger. Sovner and Hurley (1991) report that aggression may reflect a physical illness and that any initial assessment of aggression must first rule out pain, medication side effects or seizure-related mood disorder.

A population study found that 22.1% of learning-disabled people also have epilepsy (Welsh Office, 1995) compared to 0.4–1% in the general population (Chadwick, 1994). There is conflicting evidence in the literature as to whether or not epilepsy is responsible for challenging behaviour, and views have certainly changed since criminality was strongly believed to be associated with epilepsy (Lombroso, 1918). It is often reported that minor aggressive outbursts occur commonly in those with epilepsy, but they are no more common than in others who are similarly socially disadvantaged or who have suffered brain damage (Fenwick, 1989). Some studies demonstrate a higher than expected level of imprisonment compared to the non-epileptic population (e.g Gunn and Bonn, 1971), but this is more often for non-violent offending.

CONCLUSION

Diagnosis is vital in the provision of services to deaf people with challenging behaviour. However, diagnosis is dependent on cultural factors, which may not be apparent to generic clinicians who have no experience of working with deaf clients. Differential diagnosis is a complex matter, and language difficulties on either the part of the patient or the clinician will seriously impede the accuracy of diagnosis. Difficulties in providing rigorous evidence-based research compound this. Rates of misdiagnosis in deaf people have been and continue to be extremely high. Although such mistakes are usually not malevolent, they maintain an oppressive power imbalance between deaf and hearing people. Communication, as a function of mental illness and learning disability, in relation to challenging behaviour is seen alternatively as its cause, the reason for its misdiagnosis and its solution.

REFERENCES

American Psychiatric Association (1994) *Diagnostic and Statistical Manual of Mental Disorders* (4th edn.), Washington, American Psychiatric Association.

Andrews GJ (2006) Managing challenging behaviour in dementia. *British Medical Journal* 332(7544): 741.

Atkinson JR (2006) The perceptual characteristics of voice-hallucinations in deaf people: insights into the nature of subvocal thought and sensory feedback loops. *Schizophrenia Bulletin Advance Access*, http://schizophreniabulletin.oxfordjournals.org/cgi/rapidpdf/sbj063?ijkey=jPUpPjwzB1qeopt&keytype=ref, accessed 23 April 2006.

Austen S (2004) Older adults who use sign language. In Austen S, Crocker S (eds) *Deafness In Mind: Working Psychologically Across the Lifespan*, London, Whurr, pp. 329–41.

Austen S, Checinski K (2000) Addictive behaviour and deafness. In Hindley P, Kitson N (eds), *Mental Health and Deafness*, London, Whurr, pp. 232–52.

Barlow K, Grenyer B, Ilkiw-Lavalle O (2000) Prevalence and precipitants of aggression in psychiatric inpatient units. *Australian and New Zealand Journal of Psychiatry* 34(6): 967–74.

Basilier T (1964) Surdophrenia. *Acta Psychiatrica Scandinavica* 40(180): 363–72.

Bond D (2000) Mental health in children who are deaf and have multiply disabilities. In Hindley P, Kitson N (eds), *Mental Health and Deafness*, London, Whurr, pp. 127–143.

Borthwick-Duffy SA (1994) Prevalence of destructive behaviors. In Thompson T, Gray DB (eds), *Destructive Behavior in Developmental Disabilities: Diagnosis and Treatment*, Thousand Oaks, CA, SAGE, pp. 3–23.

Braden JP (1992) Intellectual assessment of deaf and hard of hearing people: a quantitative and qualitative research synthesis. *School Psychology* 21(1): 82–94.

Braden JP (1994) *Deafness, Deprivation and IQ*, London, Plenum Press.

Chadwick D (1994) Epilepsy. *Journal of Neurology, Neurosurgery and Psychiatry* 57: 264–77.

Cohen-Mansfield J, Marx MS, Rosenthal AS (1990) Dementia and agitation in nursing home residents: how are they related? *Psychology of Aging* 5(1): 3–8.

Crocker S, Edwards L (2004) Deafness and additional difficulties. In Austen S, Crocker S (eds), *Deafness in Mind: Working Psychologically with Deaf People Across the Lifespan*, London, Whurr, pp. 252–69.

Cromwell J (2005) Deafness and the art of psychometric testing. *The Psychologist* 18(12): 738–40.

Cunningham C (1982) *Down's Syndrome: An Introduction for Parents*, London, Souvenir Press.

Davidson B (2002) *Prevalence of Alcohol Use Disorders Among Deaf Psychiatric Patients*, Unpublished MSc Dissertation, University of London.

Denmark J (1966) Mental illness and early profound deafness. *British Journal of Medical Pschology* 39: 117–24.

Denmark J (1985) A study of 250 patients referred to a department of psychiatry for the deaf. *British Journal of Psychiatry*, 146: 282–86.

Dickert J (1988) Examination of bias in mental health evaluation of deaf patients. *National Association of Social Workers* 33(3): 273–4.

Dye M, Kyle J (2001) *Deaf People in the Community: Health and Disability*, Bristol, Deaf Studies Trust.

Emerson E (1995) *Challenging Behaviour*, Cambridge, Cambridge University Press.

Emerson E, Kiernan C, Alborz A, Reeves D, Mason H *et al.* (2001) The prevalence of challenging behaviours: a total population study. *Research in Developmental Disabilities* 22: 77–93.

Farroq S, Fear C (2003) Working through interpreters. *Advances in Psychiatric Treatment* 9: 104–9.

Fenwick P (1989) The nature and management of aggression in epilepsy. *Journal of Neuropsychiatry and Clinical Neuroscience* 1: 418–25.

Freeman RD, Carbin CF, Boese RJ (1981) *Can't Your Child Hear? A Guide for Those Who Care About Deaf Children, Baltimore*, University Park Press.

Graham K, Leonard, KE, Room R, Wild TC, Pihl RO *et al.* (1998) Current directions in research on understanding and preventing intoxicated aggression. *Addiction* 93(5): 659–76.

Gray A, du Feu M (2004) The causes of schizophrenia and its implications for deaf people. In Austen S, Crocker S (eds). *Deafness in Mind: Working Psychologically Across the Lifespan*, London, Whurr, pp. 206–21.

Gregory S, Bishop J, Sheldon L (1995) *Deaf People and Their Families: Developing Understanding*, Cambridge, Cambridge University Press.

Griggs M (2004) Deaf wellness explored. In Austen S, Crocker S (eds), *Deafness in Mind: Working Psychologically Across the Lifespan*, London, Whurr, pp. 115–26.

Gunn J, Bonn J (1971) Criminality and violence in epileptic prisoners. *British Journal of Psychiatry* 118(544): 337–43.

Harry B (1986) Interview, diagnostic and legal aspects in the forensic psychiatric assessments of deaf persons. *Bulletin of the American Academy of Psychiatry Law* 14(2): 147–62.

Hindley P (2000) Child and adolescent psychiatry. In Hindley P, Kitson N (eds), *Mental Health and Deafness*, London, Whurr, pp. 42–74.

Hindley P, Hill P, Bond D (1993) Interviewing deaf children, the interviewer effect: a research note. *Journal of Child Psychology and Psychiatry* 34(8): 1461–7.

Hindley P, Kitson N, Leach V (2000) Forensic psychiatry and deaf people. In Hindley P, Kitson N (eds). *Mental Health and Deafness*, London, Whurr, pp. 206–31.

Kevan F (2003) Challenging behaviour and communication difficulties. *British Journal of Learning Disabilites* 31: 75–80.

Kiernan C, Kiernan D (1994) Challenging behaviour in schools for pupils with severe learning difficulties. *Mental Handicap Research* 7: 117–210.

Kitson N, Fry R (1990) Prelingual deafness and psychiatry. *British Journal of Hospital Medicine* 244: 353–6.

Kitson N, Thacker A (2000) Adult psychiatry. In Hindley P, Kitson N (eds), *Mental Health and Deafenss*, London, Whurr, pp. 75–98.

Lane H (1993) *The Mask of Benevolence: Disabling the Deaf Community*, New York, Vintage.

Lobo A, Launer LJ , Fratiglioni L, Andersen K, Di Carlo A *et al.* (2000) Prevalence of dementia and major sub-types in Europe: a collaborative study of population based cohorts. *Neurology* 54(11 Suppl 5): S4–9.

Lombroso C (1918) *Crime: Its Causes and Remedies*, Boston, Little, Brown and Company.

Mayberry RI (2002) Cognitive development in deaf children: the interface of language and perception in neuropsychology. In Segalowitz SJ, Rapin I (eds), *Handbook of Neuropsychology* (2nd edn.), vol. 8, pt. 2, pp. 77–107.

Merck (2006) The Merck Manuals. Psychiatric Disorders. http://www.merck.com/mrkshare/mmanual/section15/chapter191/191a.jsp, accessed 26 March 2006.

O'Rourke S, Beail N (2004) Suggestibility and related concepts: implications for clinical and forensic practice with deaf people. In Austen S, Crocker S (eds), *Deafness in Mind, Working Psychologically Across the Lifespan*, London, Whurr, pp. 273–83.

Peterson CC, Siegal M (1999) Representing inner worlds: theory of mind in autistic, deaf, and normal hearing children. *Psychological Science* 10: 126–9.

Read J, Baker S (1996) *Not Just Sticks and Stones: a Survey of the Stigma, Taboos and Discrimination Experienced by People with Mental Health Problems*, London, Mind.

Reeves D, Kokoruwe B, Dobbins J, Newton V (2003) Access to primary care and Accident and Emergency departments for Deaf people. National Primary Care Research and Development Centre, University of Manchester, http://www.npcrdc.ac.uk/PublicationDetail.cfm?ID=121, accessed 23 April 2006.

Roeleveld N, Zielhuis GA, Gabreels F (1997) The prevalence of mental retardation: a critical review of recent literature. *Developmental Medicine & Child Neurology* 39(2): 125–32.

Royal National Institute for Deaf People (1998) *Breaking the Sound Barrier*, London, Royal National Institute for Deaf People.

Schildroth A (1976) *The Relationship of Nonverbal, Intelligence Test Scores to Selected Characteristics of Hearing Impaired Students*, Washington, Gallaudet College: Office of Demographic Studies.

Schlesinger HP, Meadow KP (1972) *Sound and Sign: Childhood Deafness and Mental Health*, Berkeley, CA, University of California Press.

Shapira NA, DelBello MP, Goldsmith TD, Rosenberger BM, Keck PE (1999) Evaluation of bipolar disorder in inpatients with prelingual deafness. *American Journal of Psychiatry* 156(8): 1267–9.

Sigafoos J (2000) Communication development and aberrant behaviour in children with developmental disabilities. Education and Training in Mental Retardation and Developmental Disabilities 35(2): 168–76.

Sovner R, Hurley AD (1991) The functional significance of problem behaviour: a key to effective treatment. *Habilitative Mental Healthcare Newsletter* 10: 10.

Thacker A (1991) Communication: disorder, deprivation, or discrimination? Proceedings of the Inaugural Conference of the British Society on Mental Health and Deafness. London, St George's Hospital Medial School, November 1991.

Thacker A (2001) What can we learn from the Deaf patient? In France J, Kramer S (eds), *Communication and Mental Illness: Theoretical and Practical Approaches*, London, Jessica Kingsley, pp. 251–61.

Thacker AJ (1994) Formal communication disorder: sign language in deaf people with schizophrenia. *British Journal of Psychiatry* 165(6): 818–23.

Timehin C, Timehin E (2004) Prevalence of hearing impairment in a community population of adults with learning disability: access to audiology and impact on behaviour. *British Journal of Learning Disabilities* 32: 128–32.

Vernon M, Miller K (2005) Obstacles faced by deaf people in the criminal justice system. *American Annals of the Deaf* 150(3): 283–91.

Welsh Office (1995) *Welsh Health Survey*, Cardiff, Welsh Office.

Williams C, Austen S (2000) Deafness and intellectual impairment. In Hindley P, Kitson N (eds), *Mental Health and Deafness*, London, Whurr, pp. 99–126.

World Health Organization (1992) *International Statistical Classification of Diseases and Related Health Problems*, 10th Revision, Geneva, World Health Organization.

Yeates S (1992) Have they got a hearing loss? A follow-up study of hearing in people with a mental handicap. *Mental Handicap* 20: 126–33.

Yeates S (1995) The incidence and importance of hearing loss in people with severe learning disability: the evolution of a service. *British Journal of Learning Disabilities* 23: 79–84.

PART II
Aetiology of Challenging Behaviour

5

Challenging Behaviour in the Young Deaf Child

ROSIE KENTISH

INTRODUCTION

Living with a young child can be an enriching experience for parents but few will traverse these years without the occasional sleepless night over their child's behaviour. For the deaf child, these are critical years for social and emotional development, with skills of negotiation and communication to be learnt on both sides. Although the parenting of a deaf child requires some adaptations, the fundamental parenting tasks are the same as for any other child.

This chapter looks at some of the factors related to the increased risk of behavioural difficulties in the deaf child, and at factors that underpin or undermine effective parenting. Language and communication play a central role in parents' attempts to shape their child's behaviour. Attributions and beliefs that parents hold about deafness, particularly for hearing parents of deaf children, will influence the way that they respond to their child's behaviour and can exacerbate challenging behaviour. Overly protective and indulgent parenting will not only affect the child's behaviour but can also over time affect the older child's beliefs about their responsibility for their own behaviour, the negative effects of which may endure into adulthood.

Parents who do not view deafness as a tragedy and hold a positive identity of deafness are more likely to parent effectively and insist upon socially acceptable behaviour, as with any other child.

Deafness and Challenging Behaviour: The 360° Perspective. Edited by S. Austen and D. Jeffery
© 2007 John Wiley & Sons Ltd

BEHAVIOURAL PROBLEMS IN THE YOUNG DEAF CHILD

Determining the prevalence of psychological and behavioural difficulties in the deaf child population is fraught with difficulties. The presence of additional disabilities, lack of valid assessment tools and a scarcity of mental health professionals with sufficient communication skills or experience of deafness are only some of the factors (Hindley, 1997). This may well explain why prevalence rates in the literature for mental disorders vary from 15% to 60% for children and adolescents. Nevertheless, it appears to be the case that children with hearing impairments experience the same range of mental health problems as hearing children (Bailly *et al.*, 2003).

Hearing parents of the young deaf child more commonly describe behavioural difficulties relating to sleep, overactivity and temper tantrums. Deaf children are more likely than hearing children to be described by their mothers as disobedient, restless, possessive, overly dependent and fussy (Adams and Tidwell, 1988). A number of studies have suggested greater impulsiveness in deaf and hearing-impaired children. The incidence of ADHD does not appear to be higher than for the general child population, however, with the exception of children with acquired hearing loss and/or additional disabilities (Hindley and Kroll 1998; Bailly *et al.*, 2003).

In terms of risk factors for psychological disorder in deaf children, the degree of deafness alone does not seem to be a major factor. Lack of communication skills has been identified by many researchers as being of far greater importance (Hindley, 2000), as is the presence of additional difficulties. Deaf and hearing-impaired children are approximately three times more likely to have additional difficulties such as cerebral palsy, pervasive developmental disorders, epilepsy and learning disabilities (Hindley and Roberts, 1999). Delayed development of Theory of Mind skills (the ability to understand other people's inner worlds and reflect upon one's own thoughts and feelings) is possibly associated with increased prevalence of challenging behaviour due to the child's inability to understand the world around them. Deaf children with hearing parents fare poorly in terms of Theory of Mind development compared to hearing children, as well as to deaf signing children of deaf signing parents (Russell *et al.*, 1998; Woolfe *et al.*, 2002; Peterson, 2004).

Although research is sparse, deaf children of deaf parents do not appear to have higher rates of challenging behaviour than hearing children of hearing parents (Hindley, 2000). Overall, deaf children of deaf parents are reported to attain better emotional and cognitive outcomes than do deaf children of hearing parents (Bailly *et al.*, 2003). They are also reported to have better self-image and less difficulty with impulse control (Meadow-Orlans, 1990).

LANGUAGE, COMMUNICATION AND SOCIAL DEVELOPMENT

Language plays a major role in the task of learning socially appropriate behaviour.

> As children get older, linguistic interaction becomes even more important for social and emotional development, as parents communicate social norms, behavioural rules, and the reasons for observed and imminent social and emotional events. Effective modes of parent–child and child–child communication provide for rapid and detailed transmission of social information, both implicitly and explicitly. Lack of such communication has been shown in several studies to be related to impulsive behaviour, poorer self-image, more disruptive behaviour, and an external locus of control on the part of the deaf child. (Vaccari and Marschark, 1997, pp. 798–9)

All behaviours are a form of social communication and, when language skills are limited, the chances of a child expressing their needs and feelings through what may be seen as challenging behaviour are even greater. A child's tantrum over having to wait for something may be defined as a challenging behaviour, communicating frustration or both. Without language as a means of accessing information about their world, young deaf children are more heavily dependent upon routine and consistency to understand their world: how events are connected and sequenced, that cause and effect are linked and that events or behaviours have consequences for themselves and/or for others. These skills are fundamental to the deaf child in their engagement with the social world. Absence of such skills may well underpin challenging behaviour in later years.

In deaf children of hearing parents, delay in acquiring Theory of Mind skills appears to be linked to a poor acquisition of language (Woolfe *et al.*, 2002). These skills usually develop in the preschool years and their absence may also reflect reduced life experiences. For example, interactions with family, friends and siblings that are often mediated by language, provide opportunities for learning about the mental states of others and the relationship of these states to behaviour. Delayed emotional understanding has implications for social, behavioural and cognitive development, and renders the deaf child at a disadvantage in social situations over and above those already stemming from any speech and language delay.

The consequences of impaired language and communication for parent–child interaction and management of behaviour are significant. Not only can they result in less satisfying interactions between parent and child, but they can also affect the parent's choice of style of behavioural management. Observations of mothers and deaf children's interactions in play indicate that hearing mothers tend to be overly controlling and intrusive with their deaf preschool child (Lederburg, 1993). Knutson *et al.* (2004) found that mothers of deaf children were more likely than parents of hearing children to select physical responses to child transgressions, and for the discipline to escalate if the child persisted with the transgression. In contrast to hearing children, misbehaviour more frequently leads to the deaf child being withdrawn from the situation rather than being verbally admonished. The consequences for the child of this particular behaviour-management style are that, in effect, the child has fewer opportunities to learn from past difficulties or to learn substitute behaviours that would be more acceptable. In addition, parents are demonstrating that avoidance and physical action are acceptable ways of solving difficulties (Meadow-Orlans, 1990).

The language skill and choice of the parent is inextricably linked to the language skills of the child. For deaf parents who communicate with their deaf child through sign, the language of the parent–child interaction is less problematic. The situation is different for deaf children with hearing parents who view sign with ambivalence or who are learning sign language alongside their child. Many parents feel reluctant to allow their deaf child access to sign in the belief that this threatens their best efforts to integrate the child into the hearing community. Some professionals promote this stance. The dilemma is that this may increase the risk of poor social development and behavioural difficulties in their child.

Issues of discipline, explanation of social mores, promotion of socially appropriate behaviour and the development of social understanding are all thus affected by limited language and communication (NDCS, 2003a). However, although deaf children are vulnerable, this does not mean that poor social behaviour is inevitable. Nor does it mean that parental expectations of the child's behaviour should be diminished. The essential parenting tasks remain the same but need to be approached in a different way. The implications of language and communication need to be taken into account, but are not insurmountable.

STRESS AND PARENTAL COPING

Having a child with a disability has been linked with both increased parental stress and with increased levels of behavioural difficulties (Woolfson, 2004). Stress in parents of hearing children has been linked to maternal depression (Gelfand *et al.*, 1992), insecure attachment (Jarvis and Creasey, 1991) and more negative interactive patterns between parent and child (Crnic and Greenberg, 1990). For parents of a disabled child, stress can arise from a number of factors such as increased demands upon a family's resources and visits to hospitals. Where the child is deaf, feelings of social isolation may be exacerbated by the child's limited language and communication skills, or by use of sign language, which others outside the home do not know. Behavioural problems in the child can be socially isolating.

Research into parental stress in parents of deaf and hearing-impaired children has shown conflicting results. Some research suggests that stress levels may not necessarily be higher in parents of deaf children, particularly where families have been given early intervention services. However, depending upon the type of parental stress measured, as many as 16% of these mothers may be experiencing stress that would be considered to be at a clinically significant level (Pipp-Siegel *et al.*, 2002). Parental coping and adjustment to their child's deafness reflects a complex interaction between familial socio-economic circumstances, factors within the child, the parent and the level of support provided for the family (NDCS, 2003b).

The use of social support systems is well documented as being a factor in family coping and adjustment to deafness (Pipp-Siegel *et al.*, 2002). With the recent introduction of the Neonatal Hearing Screening Programme in the UK, support should be available to families at an earlier stage. Whatever the quality and quantity of support, however, some families report finding support more useful than others. Quittner *et al.* (1990) did not find a relationship between levels of support and parental adjustment to deafness but between the parents' perceptions of that support and parental adjustment.

Psychological factors within the parent, in terms of coping strategies, are correlated with parental adjustment and with their ability to cope with the additional life stressors resulting from their child's deafness. Recent studies have begun to examine cognitive appraisal in parents of disabled children, that is the way that a particular individual assesses their life circumstances (Woolfson, 2004). Individuals vary in the extent to which they adopt a positive or negative appraisal of deafness – as a major stressor or as a welcome event. Thus, parental perceptions of deafness and their appraisal of their circumstances may be as influential as deafness itself.

PARENTAL APPRAISAL OF COMPETENCE

Despite the additional stressors and challenges, many parents cope very well with their child's deafness. For all parents, however, a sense of competence in their own parenting abilities is essential. The majority of hearing parents will have had little prior experience of deafness, and the arrival of a deaf child into their lives leaves many feeling they have entered uncharted territory, in all sorts of ways. Parenting skills they might have used if their child had been hearing may now seem invalid. There are undoubtedly new skills to be learned to effectively parent their child, for example using visual communication and facilitative interactional styles, and it is of little surprise that parents describe feeling deskilled and powerless.

In the face of their child's challenging behaviour, many parents benefit from professional support and advice around effective behavioural strategies. However, uptake of this advice is likely to be much greater if parents are helped to re-establish their sense of competency and to see that their essential parenting skills remain valid but that some adaptations to their particular child's abilities and needs is required, as with any child.

THE EFFECT ON CHALLENGING BEHAVIOUR OF PARENTAL APPRAISAL OF DEAFNESS

Woolfson's (2004) theoretical model of disability-related child-behaviour problems examines psychosocial factors of disability and impairment and the influence of negative societal views of disability upon parents' ability to manage their child's behaviour.

THE MEDICAL MODEL OF DEAFNESS

As we move into the 21st century, the potential and contributions of deaf people in society have increased considerably, and British Sign

Language (BSL) has been recognised as the fourth native language of the UK. However, Woolfson (2004) considers the prevailing societal views of disability as being one of tragedy – for both the parent and the child. Viewed from the medical model of disability, predominant within Western society, disability is seen as a problem located within the individual, as with an illness. From this starting point, a focus of intervention that alleviates both the impairment and the disability of deafness by maximizing the child's ability to speak and hear 'normally' make sense (Schwartz, 1996). Hearing aids or a cochlear implant thus offer the hope of restoring the hearing child that parents had expected.

Parental beliefs about disability will depend in part upon their own personal life experiences but will also reflect these wider societal beliefs. When prevailing societal beliefs about disability are largely negative, this has corresponding implications for how parents will respond to their child's diagnosis, for the decisions that they make on their child's behalf and for their beliefs about child rearing and discipline.

THE CULTURAL MODEL OF DEAFNESS

In contrast, the cultural model regards Deaf people as belonging to a linguistic and cultural minority group (Austen and Coleman, 2004). It views deafness as an alternative way of being, of living life to the full through a visual world rather than as an audiological deficit. As a group, members of the Deaf community present a strong challenge to the stance that deafness is a disability. In contrast to hearing parents, many Deaf parents are less likely to see their child's deafness as a tragedy, but welcome the arrival of a deaf child, with whom they will share a cultural identity and language (Feher-Prout, 1996).

For the hearing parent of a deaf child, the Deaf cultural perspective can be liberating, offering a more affirmative view of being deaf. Alternatively, it can be experienced as negating their sense of loss and grief. The situation is complex, as Gregory (2004) points out:

> The notion of a strong Deaf community rather than offering a positive solution to hearing mothers, presents a further dilemma. In acknowledging that their child is Deaf, they are in a sense losing their child to a different language and cultural group, for part of child rearing is the sharing and developing of a common culture. (Gregory, 2004)

IMPLICATIONS OF PARENTAL APPRAISAL OF DEAFNESS FOR BEHAVIOUR MANAGEMENT

In day-to-day reality, the dual positions of the medical model and the deaf cultural model are not mutually exclusive, and most parents will find themselves positioned somewhere between the two on the various different issues. Extreme positions are rarely helpful. Effective parenting acknowledges both the special needs of the deaf child, as well as the need to be treated as any other child. When difficulties arise, however, and behaviour becomes problematic and challenging, one aspect of professional intervention is to consider parental beliefs and cognitions around deafness and communication, and perceptions of the locus of responsibility for difficult behaviour.

CHALLENGING BEHAVIOUR AS AN INEVITABLE CONSEQUENCE OF DEAFNESS

Woolfson's (2004) model hypothesises that, according to the medical model, parents are likely to view their child's behaviour through the 'lens' of the impairment, in this case, deafness. In the same way that deafness is inherent to the child, so difficult behaviour may come to be seen as an inevitable and unalterable part of deafness. The implications of this are that parents may then believe they have no choice but to tolerate problematic behaviour, leaving them feeling helpless and deskilled. The parenting strategies that they would normally have used no longer seem appropriate, or seem harder to implement, when faced by challenging behaviour. Furthermore, hearing parents are less likely to feel that implementing a behavioural approach will result in positive change. The author argues that the Deaf parent, in the absence of a view that deafness is a disability, will be advantaged in their parenting in that they are likely to construe any behavioural difficulties as typical for the child's developmental stage rather than as a consequence of deafness. Support for this position comes from the finding that Deaf parents rate their experience on a range of communicative, behavioural and developmental parenting tasks as far less difficult than hearing parents (NDCS, 2003b). This may be due to a number of factors: familiarity with deafness, ease of communication with the child or the statistical likelihood of the child not having additional disabilities. However, in the author's opinion, it is the Deaf parents' differing expectations of and explanations for their child's behaviour that is potentially different and pivotal.

The alternative scenario, however, whereby parents fail to acknowledge the developmental and behavioural correlates of deafness, is not without its challenges. For if the parent does not see behavioural difficulties as part of their child's disability, they are more likely to feel anger towards the child. In a study of mothers of disabled children Chavira *et al.* (2000) found that most of the mothers in their sample did not perceive their disabled children as being responsible for their problematic behaviour, but those who did experienced negative emotions towards their child. In hearing children, attributing responsibility solely to the child for problematic behaviour has been linked to greater stress, more negative emotional reactions in the parent and to harsher punishment (Graham *et al.*, 2001).

Woolfson (2004) advises that professional intervention should be aimed at affecting the parents' causal beliefs about their child's disability (in this case deafness) and to help parents to see their child's behavioural difficulties as typical problems faced by any parents of a child at that developmental stage. She reports that:

> This empowered parents to implement caregiving strategies with which they were familiar, rather than feeling that parenting a disabled child required them to learn new and special techniques. (Woolfson, 2004, p. 4)

DEAFNESS AS A 'TRAGEDY' FOR WHICH THE CHILD NEEDS TO BE COMPENSATED

A further consequence of seeing deafness as a disability may well be that parents feel a responsibility to compensate the child for the 'tragedy' of being deaf. Within a clinical setting, it is not uncommon to see parents whose natural feelings of protectiveness have become magnified and who seek to compensate their child for any distress and hardship they have experienced or will experience as a result of their deafness. As a result, they make greater allowances for their child and find it harder to instil appropriate boundaries for behaviour. They are reluctant to discipline or upset their child. A contrary view, in which deafness is seen neither as a tragedy nor as a disability, and where a positive identity of deafness is held, is more likely to result in parenting that insists upon socially acceptable behaviour, as with any other child. Tackling parental perceptions and behaviours in the early years may thus have a lifetime of benefits.

THE OVERPROTECTION OF THE DEAF CHILD: BELIEFS ABOUT DEPENDENCY

When communication between parent and child is dramatically reduced, parents tend to become more protective and feel that their child needs more supervision than a hearing child (Meadow-Orlans, 1990). Parents who take on the role of protector seek to shelter their child both socially and emotionally from awkward situations. For example, where a child might need to interact with people with whom they have difficulty communicating, the parents may act as interpreter and negotiator on the child's behalf. By acting as the child's intermediary with the outside world, they will have greater difficulty in separating from their child and feel anxious that their child cannot manage without them. Such protectiveness must be balanced with the necessary parental task of fostering independence and coping skills in the child.

Parental overprotectiveness is well intentioned, shielding the child in the short term from difficult life experiences. Its consequences over the longer term are not so beneficial and are likely to result in a child who is passive, dependent and less mature socially. When parents have a belief system that sees difficult behaviours as an inherent part of deafness and its associated language difficulties, it is possible that this becomes internalised by the deaf child. The child will similarly find it difficult to accept responsibility for their own behaviour and are likely to locate the responsibility for behaviour or personal difficulties either within others or within the deafness itself. The deaf child will likely continue to grow into a deaf adult who continues to deny personal responsibility.

Again, deaf parents appear to be at an advantage. Indeed, Meadow-Orlans (1990) observes that deaf parents tend to grant independence at a younger age, and that 'deaf parents of deaf children appear to be less anxious about their deaf pre-schoolers' abilities to navigate within their neighbourhood independently, about environmental dangers, and generally about their ability to care for themselves' (p. 290–1).

CONCLUSION

Parenting any child can be challenging, and parenting a deaf child may be even more so. There are inevitably changes in parental style when a child lives in a predominantly visual world. The task of parenting a deaf child is complex, but viewing the world from a visual perspective brings forth rich and varied approaches to parenting and interaction, emphasising the importance of non-verbal behavioural cues and visually and physically oriented interactions to support communication.

Parenting style, stress levels and beliefs about their own competency can influence the presence or absence of challenging behaviour in a child. Likewise, the parent's beliefs about the causes of their child's challenging behaviour will affect their parenting choices, which in turn affect their management of the behaviour. The choices, beliefs and behaviours of the parent have a bearing not only on the behaviour of their child but also on the adult they will grow into.

Deaf children of hearing parents appear to have a higher incidence of challenging behaviour than deaf children of deaf parents. This is only partly explained by the lower incidence of additional difficulties in deaf children of deaf parents. Woolfson (2004) suggests that negative perceptions of a child's disability by society or the parent increase the chance that the parent will tolerate the child's challenging behaviour, thereby increasing its likelihood. An alternative stance, whereby parents fail to acknowledge the disabling aspects of deafness and its consequences for language and communication, and for social and cognitive development, is equally problematic.

Parents, deaf or hearing, who hold a more affirmative view of deafness and do not see deafness as inherently linked to socially unacceptable behaviour are more likely to actively promote their children's independence and self-reliance. Likewise, such parents will have high expectations of their deaf child's behaviour and use appropriate discipline and boundary setting with the child. Research using deaf parents who are less likely to regard their child's deafness as a tragedy is still unfortunately sparse.

The central role of language and communication for social development and Theory of Mind development is clear. Ensuring optimum communication, by whatever means, whether visual, verbal or nonverbal is essential. In children who use sign language, the sign language competence of their parents is also of consequence. The Deaf cultural model offers a more affirmative view of deafness and of sign as a valid language, but hearing parents will also have concerns about how their culturally Deaf child (and future working age child) will learn to negotiate the hearing world.

Professional intervention should be aimed at the level of parental belief and perception. Parental beliefs about the consequences of deafness appear to affect the degree of overprotectiveness and indulgence.

The dangers inherent in adopting a seemingly more protective and tolerant position can have damaging consequences for the deaf child that may last into adulthood, affecting all aspects of life, ultimately affecting mental health and well-being.

Political positioning aside, what is most important of all is that the child retains status as a child first. The deaf child has the same parenting needs as any child: is expected and supported to develop positive social behaviour, independence and the skills necessary to negotiate the social world. If parents and professionals retain high expectations of the deaf child's behaviour, with the management, interventions and consequences that hearing children are afforded, the child has the opportunity of appropriate social growth and development in the critical early years. Tackling parental perceptions and behaviours in the early years may thus have a lifetime of benefits.

REFERENCES

Adams JW, Tidwell R (1988) Parents' perceptions regarding the discipline of their hearing-impaired children. *Childcare, Health and Development* 14(4): 265–73.

Austen S, Coleman E (2004) Controversy in deafness: Animal Farm meets Brave New World. In Austen S, Crocker C (eds), *Deafness in Mind: Working Psychologically with Deaf People Across the Lifespan*, London, Whurr Publishers, pp. 3–20.

Bailly D, Dechoulydelenclave MB, Lauwerier L (2003) Hearing impairment and psychopathological disorders in children and adolescents: review of the literature. *Encephale* 29(4 pt1): 329–37.

Chavira V, Lopez S, Blacher J, Shapiro J (2000) Latina mothers' attributions, emotions, and reactions to the problem behaviors of their children with developmental disabilities. *Journal of Child Psychology and Psychiatry* 41(2): 245–52.

Crnic K, Greenberg MT (1990) Minor parenting stresses with young children. *Child Development* 61(5): 1628–37.

Feher-Prout T (1996) Stress and coping in families with deaf children. *Journal of Deaf Studies and Deaf Education* 1(3): 155–65.

Gelfand DM, Teti DM, Fox CE (1992) Sources of parenting stress for depressed and nondepressed mothers of infants. *Journal of Clinical Child Psychology* 21: 262–72.

Graham S, Weiner B, Cobb M, Henderson T (2001) An attributional analysis of child abuse among low-income African American mothers. *Journal of Social and Clinical Psychology* 20(2): 233–57.

Gregory S (2004) Challenging motherhood: mothers and their deaf children. http://www.deafnessatbirth.org.uk/, accessed 23 March 2006.

Hindley PA (1997) Psychiatric aspects of hearing impairments. *Journal of Child Psychology and Psychiatry* 38(1): 101–17.

Hindley PA (2000) Child and adolescent psychiatry. In Hindley PA, Kitson N (eds), *Mental Health and Deafness*, London, Whurr, pp. 42–74.

Hindley P, Kroll L (1998) Theoretical and epidemiological aspects of attention deficit and overactivity in deaf children. *Journal of Deaf Studies and Education* 3(1): 64–72.

Hindley P, Roberts C (1999) Practitioner review: the assessment and treatment of deaf children with psychiatric disorders. *Journal of Child Psychology and Psychiatry* 40(2): 151–67.

Jarvis PA, Creasey GL (1991) Parenting stress, coping, and attachment in families with an 18-month-old infant. *Infant Behaviour and Development* 14: 383–95.

Knutson JF, Johnson CR, Sullivan PM (2004) Disciplinary choices of mothers of deaf children and mothers of normally hearing children. *Child Abuse and Neglect* 28(9): 925–37.

Lederberg AR (1993) The impact of deafness on mother-child and peer relationships. In Marschark M, Clark MD (eds), *Psychological Perspectives on Deafness*. Hillsdale, NJ, Lawrence Erlbaum, pp. 93–119.

Meadow-Orlans KP (1990) Research on developmental aspects of deafness. In Moores DF, Meadow-Orlans KP (eds), *Educational and Developmental Aspect of Deafness*, Washington, Gallaudet University Press, pp. 283–98.

NDCS (2003a) *Parenting and Deaf Children: A Psychosocial Literature Based Framework*, London, National Deaf Children's Society.

NDCS (2003b) *Parenting and Deaf Children: Report on the Needs Assessment Study Undertaken as Part of the NDCS Toolkit Development Project*, London, National Deaf Children's Society.

Peterson CC (2004) Theory of Mind development in oral deaf children with cochlear implants or conventional hearing aids. *Journal of Child Psychology and Psychiatry* 45(6): 1096–106.

Pipp-Siegel S, Sedey A, Yoshinaga-Itano C (2002) Predictors of parental stress in mothers of young children with hearing loss. *Journal of Deaf Studies and Deaf Education* 7(1): 1–17.

Quittner A, Glueckauf R, Jackson D (1990) Chronic parenting stress: moderating versus mediating effects of social support. *Journal of Personality and Social Psychology* 59(6): 1266–78.

Russell PA, Hosie CD, Gray CD, Scott C, Hunter N (1998) The development of theory of mind in deaf children. *Journal of Child Psychology and Psychiatry* 39(6): 903–10.

Schwartz S (1996) *Choices in Deafness: A Parent's Guide to Communication Options* (2nd edition), Bethesda, MD, Woodbine House Inc.

Vaccari C, Marschark M (1997) Communication between parents and deaf children: implications for social-emotional development. *Journal of Child Psychology and Psychiatry* 38(7): 793–801.

Woolfe T, Want SC, Siegal M (2002) Signposts to development: theory of mind in deaf children. *Child Development* 73(3): 768–78.

Woolfson L (2004) Family well-being and disabled children: a psychosocial model of disability-related child behaviour problems. *British Journal of Health Psychology* 9(pt 1): 1–13.

6

Neuropsychological, Behavioural and Linguistic Factors in Challenging Behaviour in Deaf People

ROBIN PAIJMANS

INTRODUCTION

From the perspective of the principles of functional behaviour, challenging behaviour can be seen as a maladaptive coping response resulting from a disruption in normal cognitive processing. Functional communication models conceptualise challenging behaviour similarly as an attempt at communication with impaired communication ability. As such, people who experience a disruption in their cognitive processes and/or communication difficulties are more likely to exhibit challenging behaviour.

Deaf people are more likely to suffer concomitant neurological damage or learning disability. Moreover, they often suffer language developmental delays consequent to growing up in a predominantly hearing, non-deaf supportive environment and experience extensive difficulties in communicating in such settings. As such, deaf people may be more vulnerable to exhibiting behaviour that is perceived as 'challenging'. In particular, the development of language (or the absence thereof) may play a crucial role in this.

Deafness and Challenging Behaviour: The 360° Perspective. Edited by S. Austen and D. Jeffery
© 2007 John Wiley & Sons Ltd

CHALLENGING BEHAVIOUR

Challenging behaviours can range from physical or verbal aggression, destructive behaviour, absconding, agitation and (sexual) disinhibition to confabulation, acting on delusions and behaviour inappropriate to the social context in which it occurs. Xeniditis *et al.* (2001) point out that 'challenging behaviour' is a descriptive (rather than defining) concept that is largely socially constructed, and therefore its definition is subject to social norms and values, and service-delivery patterns. Depending on the context in which it occurs and the attribution of its causal factors, challenging behaviour may, for instance, not come to the attention of social, educational or healthcare services but may be dealt with within the penal system instead. Some challenging behaviour may not come to the attention of any services at all but be managed within a supportive community or normalised and tolerated within certain social environments or contexts (e.g. drunken disinhibited behaviour in the context of nights out drinking with peers), while it definitely is not in others (e.g. drunken disinhibited behaviour in the workplace).

CAUSAL FACTORS IN CHALLENGING BEHAVIOUR

It is well known that challenging behaviour is particularly associated with learning disability and brain injury. Detailed overviews of challenging behaviour in people with learning disabilities and in people with acquired brain injury are provided by Allen (2000) and Benson Yody *et al.* (2000) respectively. Studies show that, typically, the prevalence of challenging behaviour increases with the severity of cognitive disability (Borthwick-Duffy, 1994; Davidson *et al.*, 1994). This is perhaps not surprising as effective self-regulation and goal-directed behaviour involve the cooperation of a range of sophisticated cognitive functions, all of which can be affected by a disruption in brain function. Challenging behaviour has also been cited to be more prevalent in those with communication difficulties (e.g. Chamberlain *et al.*, 1993; Emerson, 1995; Schroeder *et al.*, 1978; Chung *et al.*, 1995; Sigafoos, 2000). There is a significant overlap in the two problems. In a detailed review of communication difficulties in the learning disabled, van der Gaag (1998) notes that estimates of the prevalence of communication problems in the learning-disabled population in the UK range from 50% to 89%. Hallas *et al.* (1982) comment that communication difficulties are the commonest and least treated disability amongst people with learning disabilities.

THE RELATIONSHIP BETWEEN CHALLENGING BEHAVIOUR AND DEAFNESS

DEAFNESS AND COGNITIVE IMPAIRMENT

In deafness, the overlapping problems of cognitive impairment/learning disability and communication difficulty are also prominent. Deafness is not necessarily a solitary condition; depending on its biological causal or contributing factors, it can be accompanied by impairments such as visual or cognitive deficits (e.g. Usher's syndrome) or structural heart defects and other organ dysfunction or malformation (e.g. trisomy 13 syndrome, multiple lentigines syndrome). Various non-genetic causes of deafness can cause damage to other organs including the brain (e.g. hypoxia, prenatal exposure to infectious disease) and adversely affect subsequent normal brain development to result in permanent learning disability. Approximately 30% to 40% of children who are deaf or hard of hearing may have one or more other developmental disabilities or neurological conditions such as learning disabilities, cerebral palsy or epilepsy (Crocker and Edwards, 2004). The 1993 reference issue of the *American Annals of the Deaf* reports learning disabilities as the largest co-occurring disability at a prevalence of 9%, with the prevalence of other intellectual problems following closely at 8% and co-occurrence rate of emotional/behavioural problems at 4% (Craig and Craig, 1993).

Research on the cognitive development of non-learning-disabled profoundly prelingually deaf people compared to their hearing counterparts is equivocal. Methodological difficulties in cognitive assessment abound, given that most tests and their administration procedures are standardised on a hearing population and their interpretation in use on a deaf population is often a matter of professional judgement by the individual clinician. The complexities of cognitive assessment of the deaf have been extensively explored by Braden (1992; 1994). Nevertheless, profound deafness in itself is known to affect cognitive and psychosocial development, particularly through the lack of access to language and through social isolation. This relationship is quite complex, being mediated by variables such as the onset and degree of deafness, hearing status and signing proficiency of the parents, access to Deaf environments in general and educational setting and approach (Mayberry, 2002).

DEAFNESS AND COMMUNICATION DIFFICULTIES

It is obvious that deafness will also result in communication difficulties. Although sophisticated sign languages exist, 90% of deaf children are born to hearing parents, the vast majority of whom do not learn how to sign. As such, the first exposure to a functional language may only be in a deaf educational setting, well past the first four to five years of the child's life that are critical in terms of language acquisition. As a consequence, deaf children are often far behind in terms of vocabulary and language comprehension (Mayberry, 2002), even though they perform equal to their hearing peers when enrolled in a language intervention programme as early as at eleven months of age (e.g. Moeller, 2000). This language developmental delay affects the acquisition of reading and writing skills also; the mean English literacy of deaf high-school graduates is at the 4.5 grade level (Holt, 1993). To add to these communication challenges, even if a deaf child grows up in a deaf supportive environment, the world at large is not. The vast majority of people do not sign and often no special communication provisions are made for deaf people in key areas of society such as health and social care, education and the law.

It therefore follows that the relationship between challenging behaviour and deafness can be considered in terms of the overlapping areas of cognitive impairment and communication difficulties (Figure 6.1), which this chapter will address. Any intervention in challenging behaviour in a deaf person requires an understanding of those areas and their interaction. Needless to say, very little is written about challenging behaviour in deaf people specifically; as such this chapter attempts to adapt to the deaf population what is known about the causality of challenging behaviour in hearing people.

DEFINITIONS

The terminology used in this chapter needs to be briefly clarified. With 'learning disability' is meant any cognitive, neurological or psychological disorder that impedes the ability to learn, especially one that interferes with the ability to learn sophisticated cognitive skills and language

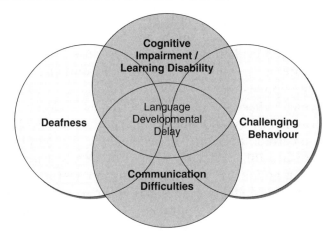

Figure 6.1 The relationship between deafness and challenging behaviour

skills. In the United States, the term 'mental retardation' may be more commonly used. Cognitive impairment can be permanent or temporary. In the former case, it may have congenital or hereditary causes, be the result of brain injury acquired at birth or later in life or be the result of prolonged physiological or psychological developmental deprivation. Cognitive functioning can be temporarily disrupted through mental or physical illness, concussion or a disturbance of normal physiological processes in the human body, such as fever, intoxication, dehydration, malnutrition or organ failure. A cognitive delay differs from a cognitive deficit in that in the former further development is possible and a level of functioning can eventually be attained that is precluded in the latter.

CHALLENGING BEHAVIOUR AND COGNITIVE IMPAIRMENT/LEARNING DISABILITY

The most influential cognitive theory of challenging behaviour has been based on the functional behavioural principles of **positive** and **negative reinforcement**. Skinner (1953) first introduced the principle that behaviour is the result of an *interaction* between the organism and its environment, that it is **purposeful** and **goal-directed** within that environment and is either **reinforced** or **extinguished** by its consequences. At its simplest, these relationships are expressed in the ABC model of behaviour: Antecedent triggers Behaviour, which results in Consequences. If the consequences are favourable, the behaviour is reinforced and more likely to occur in response to similar circumstances in future; if the consequences are unfavourable, the behaviour is extinguished and less likely to occur in future.

Exactly which behaviour (of many alternatives) an antecedent triggers is determined by the individual's interpretation of the antecedent and their perceived repertoire of available behavioural responses, which in turn are influenced by what they have learned from past experience. This notion is reflected explicitly in Lazarus and Folkman's Primary Appraisal Model (Lazarus and Folkman, 1984) in which the individual makes a **primary appraisal** of a stressor (resulting in an immediate emotional arousal response such as fear, anger, alarm, frustration, distress), followed by a **secondary appraisal** of the controllability of the stressor and coping resources available.

Whether the consequence or outcome of a behavioural response serves as reinforcement or extinction of that behaviour is again entirely dependent on the individual's appraisal of the outcome as more or less favourable than what they perceive might have happened if they had

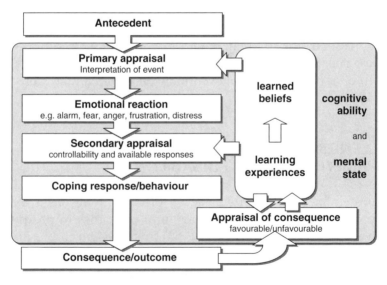

Figure 6.2 Appraisal model of behaviour (adapted from Lazarus and Folkman, 1984)

not responded in this way. In doing so, they again refer to their previously learned beliefs and past experience. Moreover, the present sequence of Antecendent → Behaviour → Consequence constitutes a learning experience in itself, which modifies learned beliefs to reinforce or extinguish the current behaviour. This whole appraisal and learning process occurs against the backdrop of the person's cognitive faculties and present mental state (Figure 6.2).

The complexity of the above process emphasises how important cognitive functioning and mental state are in the generation of functional behaviour. It also emphasises how appraisal of the appropriateness and consequences of behaviour is a very subjective matter. In the context of challenging behaviour, what may be seen as an undesirable, unpleasant or even quite harmful outcome to an observer (or recipient) of the behaviour may be perceived as relatively favourable to the person exhibiting it, compared to the possible outcome that might have resulted if they had responded in a different way. Being shouted at may be experienced as more favourable than being ignored; being forcibly removed from a social situation may be experienced as more favourable than feeling overwhelmed by it.

CHALLENGING BEHAVIOUR AS DELIBERATE OR AUTOMATIC RESPONSE

Given the fundamentally purposeful and goal-directed nature of behaviour and the cognitive processes involved in its generation, it seems logical to regard challenging behaviour as a product of purely rational insight and conscious choice; **purposefulness** is equated with **intentionality**. This can cause enormous frustration and anger in carers and staff alike, who may feel exasperated by the distressing or destructive behaviour for which they are unable to elicit a rational explanation from the offender, and which they are unable to change despite many attempts at explaining why it is unacceptable or distressing. Sooner or later, carers and staff may conclude that, given the apparent purposefulness of the offending behaviour, it must be intentional, and that the offender is simply uncaring and unwilling to change, whereupon feelings of anger and blame ensue. Alternatively, they may hold the view that challenging behaviour is the entirely unintentional, random product of a person who is out of control, and therefore that it has no purpose or logic and defies any attempts at understanding, prediction or change, that it is something to be passively endured or to be contained by any means possible but is beyond influence or comprehension.

CONSCIOUS VS. AUTOMATIC PROCESSING AND REGULATED VS. UNREGULATED BEHAVIOUR

Since essentially no behaviour is a purely random act, the question inevitably arises what else can produce purposeful behaviour, if not only conscious and deliberate intent. The cognitive psychological models of automatic vs. conscious information processing (e.g. Posner and Snyder, 1975; Dixon, 1981) and regulated vs. unregulated behaviour (discussed in detail by Brewin, 1993) offer a possible explanation.

Conscious processing is flexible and deliberate, but also slow and effortful and easily disrupted by other stimuli competing for attention. It is limited in capacity by the conscious attention span, which means that it must be selective in what sensory information to process. Conscious processing produces **regulated** behaviour that is intentional, insightful, flexible and adaptable to changing circumstances. Automatic processing, on the other hand, is fast, rigid, requires minimal attention and may happen instinctually, without conscious intention or aware-ness. It is influenced mainly by the salience of stimuli and their fre-quency or co-occurrence. It produces **unregulated** behaviour that is relatively reflex-like, automatic, simple and stereotyped, and occurs in direct response to specific environmental triggers. Because of a lack of conscious deliberation and intent, the individual may not be aware of this behaviour. However, this lack of intentionality does not mean that unregulated behaviour is not purposeful; there is an evolutionary rationale behind this arrangement. Emotional reactions can generate the physiological arousal and mental alertness required to adequately cope with important or potentially threatening events, and they allow us to respond quickly and effectively to any sudden, unexpected threat, where conscious deliberation is far too slow in responding to the situ-ation (e.g. jumping clear of danger). Immediate, instinctive reacting may mean the difference between life and death. Learned automatic behavioural routines allow us to function smoothly in many daily tasks, allowing us to direct our limited conscious processing capacity to more challenging problems that require it. As such, there is a definite functional and survival value in automatic instinctual behaviours supplementing (and occasionally hijacking) our conscious, intentional behaviour.

In the context of Folkman and Lazarus' Primary Appraisal Model, the primary-appraisal process can be regarded as predominantly gov-erned by automatic cognitive processing, and the resulting initial emotional response as a predominantly unregulated reaction. In the secondary-appraisal process, on the other hand, conscious, deliberate cognitive processing normally plays a dominant role with the resulting coping response being characterised by (self-)regulated behaviour. The postulated mechanism that enables the normally functioning person to fluently manage these two modes of cognitive processing and behaviour is called 'executive function' (Shallice, 1988; Baddeley, 1991). The basic concept, developed by Norman and Shallice (1980), is that a 'Central Executive' or 'Supervisory Attentional System' allows the person to shift attention flexibly, inhibiting automatic, unregulated responses and organising and producing regulated, intentional and goal-directed behaviour (including problem-solving, planning, execution, goal-directed and self-monitoring and social interaction) as appropriate to the environmental demands. Without this executive function, people would simply respond to environmental triggers and cues instinctively, with various possible actions and behavioural responses competing amongst themselves for execution. Given that automatic processing is fast and does not require conscious attention, unregulated responses will generally win this race unless they are inhibited by the Central Executive, which allows conscious regulated responses to be executed instead. Thus, executive functions have an important role in inhibiting initial automatic emotional reactions and regulating the complex cognitive processes that allow a person to deliberate and execute the most appropriate coping responses with intent. If this executive process is disrupted, coping responses are more likely to be unregulated reflex-like emotional reactions than intentional and considered flexible responses (Figure 6.3).

Neuroanatomy reveals discrete parts of the brain involved with automatic and conscious processing and associated unregulated and regulated behaviour. However, although 'Central Executive' or executive functions are often referred to as a single controlling entity/function, there is in fact no single brain structure that corresponds to them, and they are best regarded as a collective term for a range of processes located in the frontal lobes of the brain, which converge on a general concept of control functions (Parkin, 1998; Stuss and Alexander, 2000). These complex higher brain functions are much more susceptible to disruption than more basic reflex-like processes. Therefore, in cases where cognition has been impaired, and in moments of distress and increased emotional arousal, consciously deliberated behaviour is more likely to be disrupted and displaced by unregulated automatic reactions. Being more primitive, inflexible responses are less likely to

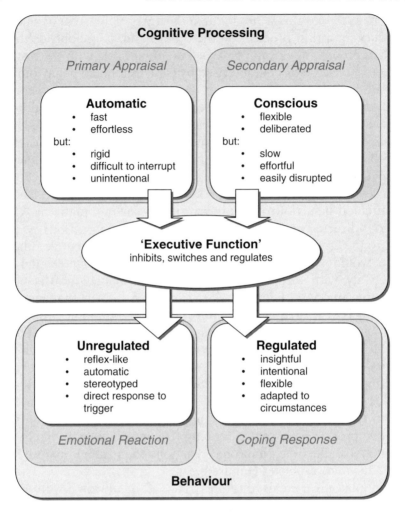

Figure 6.3 Conscious vs. unconscious processing and regulated vs. unregulated behaviour

be appropriate to the situation and more likely to constitute what would generally be regarded as challenging behaviour. Moreover, as such responses tend to be unintentional and mediated by automatic cognitive processes that occur mainly outside the person's conscious awareness, they may find it difficult to explain their behaviour in retrospect. Morris (1981), indeed, observes that people are more accurate in explaining **intended** actions than **non-intended** actions, and in the common language there are many expressions describing this phenomenon to explain apparently irrational behaviour: 'he was overcome by emotion', 'reason abandoned her', 'he got carried away', 'she acted on impulse' etc.

CHALLENGING BEHAVIOUR IN A COMMUNICATIVE CONTEXT

Carr and Durand (1994) note that challenging behaviour occurs mainly in a social context, and is designed to either draw or escape attention. In that context, challenging behaviour has the very specific purpose of communication. This has led to the **functional communication** model that challenging behaviour may occur if a more effective or appropriate form of communication is not available to the person exhibiting this behaviour. It is an attempt at coping within the constraints of one's communication difficulties with a (communicatively) challenging environment.

This perspective shifts the focus of disability from inside the person exhibiting challenging behaviour to the social barriers in the environment and from a medical model of impairment or a functional model of activity limitation to a social-inclusion model of participation restriction. People without any impairment are more capable of adjusting their communication than the person with cognitive impairment or communication difficulties; as such, family members and staff need to learn to adjust their communication accordingly to meet the person at his or her level (McConkey et al., 1999). However, in an insightful article Kevan (2003) points out that, although people may be aware of a service user's **expressive** communication difficulties because these are readily observable, his or her **receptive** communication difficulties are often underestimated at best, or disregarded at worst. Bradshaw (2001), for instance, compared staff reports of communication with learning-disabled service users with video recordings of such interactions and found that staff tended to underestimate their own use of verbal communication and overestimate their own use of non-verbal communication. The findings also indicated a mismatch between the reported level of understanding of the service user and the level of complexity of the language used. Staff appeared unable to adapt their communication to the abilities of the service user, and an average of 45% of communicative acts exceeded the reported understanding skills of the individual. Banat et al. (2002) asked members of staff to estimate their clients' comprehension of sentences at different levels of difficulty.

These estimates were subsequently compared with actual test results obtained from the clients. Differences between estimates and actual scores increased with the difficulty of the sentences. At the highest level of difficulty, staff consistently overestimated the client's ability, while both under- and overestimation occurred at the lower levels. Consequently, much behaviour that is regarded as challenging may in fact arise from confusion and misunderstanding caused simply by poor communication.

A large proportion of challenging behaviour has been observed to be an attempt to escape the situation, and this has been attributed to the aversion to certain tasks or demands in terms of their unfamiliarity or difficulty. Kevan (2003), however, proposes that as task difficulty increases so may its verbal instruction and that the aversion experienced may in fact not be to the difficulty and demands of the task but to the confusion and demands of the communication associated with it. In this context, challenging behaviour may be an attempt at escaping confusing or conflicting communication.

CHALLENGING BEHAVIOUR IN A LANGUAGE DEVELOPMENTAL DEPRIVATION CONTEXT

It is obvious that language acquisition and development affect communication ability. However, language also has an important role in the development of reasoning and concept formation, and in providing a framework within which to identify and make sense of one's experiences and emotions. Hermelin and O'Connor (1964), for instance, suggest that the developing infant goes through stages during which first visceral and introceptive sensations are dominant, superseded gradually by tactile and kinaesthetic sensations, followed by auditory and visual sensations. Subsequently, *meaning* rather than modality of the sensation determines its hierarchical significance. Luria (1961) emphasises the role of language in this process when he argues that the second signalling system of meaning and language comes to dominate the first signalling system of sensory input. On the basis of a controlled study of twins, Luria and Yudovich (1971) drew the conclusion that with the advent of speech acquisition the mental life of the twins changed drastically and abruptly. Changes in their ability to plan and execute planned behaviour occurred, which Luria and Yudovich argue could only be attributed to the influence of their burgeoning language system. As a child develops language, it acquires the cognitive tools to start naming, reflecting on and reasoning about what it perceives. It develops an internal dialogue: an intra-psychological tool for regulating thought and behaviour. Thus, language becomes not just a tool for communication but also a framework for meaningfully filtering and organising the multitude of sensory stimuli of the world and one's experiences in it, and for reasoning and planning behaviour. It is this merging of language and cognition that transforms children's minds and allows for the development of higher, uniquely human, cognitive functions such as planning, executive functioning and behavioural self-regulation (Vygotsky, 1962; Berk, 1992).

Obvious parallels can be drawn between these models, and the aforementioned models of conscious, deliberated processing vs. unconscious automatic processing and regulated vs. unregulated behaviour, with Luria's first signalling system involving automatic responding to environmental stimuli (triggers) and the second signalling system of meaning and language involving conscious deliberation and planned behaviour. It is important, then, to consider how, through its impact on language development, deafness affects cognitive development and behaviour. As Mayberry puts it:

> Can the child develop 'inner thought' or working memory without the ability to hear? Consider sign language. Can sign language foster the same kinds of abstract mental development and complex thought as speech? Now consider an even more complex situation, namely, the cognitive development of children who grow up with little or no exposure to any language in any form, be it signed or spoken, as a simple consequence of being born deaf. What are the effects of such linguistic and social isolation on the child's development of a mental life? (Mayberry, 2002, p. 71)

THE IMPORTANCE OF LANGUAGE IN DEVELOPING APPROPRIATE BEHAVIOUR

Luria and Yudovich (1971) assert that the internal dialogue that is facilitated by language plays an important role in the self-regulation of behaviour.

> By subordinating himself to the adult's verbal orders the child acquires a system of these verbal instructions and gradually begins to utilize them for the regulation of his own behaviour. (Luria and Yudovich, 1971, pp. 13–14)

In this view, it is through language that the external control of behaviour by threat of punishment is internalised, to become self-control via the self-reflective concepts of shame, guilt and embarrassment. According to Luria and Yudovitch (1971) and Vygotsky (1962), it is through language that children master their own behaviour.

Interaction and communication with other people plays an important role in this process, as it establishes a consensus of concepts and frameworks within which one's own experiences and behaviour are interpreted and reflected upon. A language shared with others is important not only for making sense of the world but also for an understanding of the world from an other's point of view. A shared language establishes a shared framework by which we can communicate our thoughts, feelings and needs to others in a meaningful way, and are able to understand the thoughts, feelings and needs that other people may convey to us. It also enables us to generate a consensus on how to view situations and events, and on the appropriateness or inappropriateness of certain behaviours in those circumstances. It enables us to imitate the appropriate behaviour of others by mapping their actions, motivations and thoughts onto our own.

Therefore, Theory of Mind (the ability to consider others' thinking, and that this can differ from one's own) is a prerequisite for the effective socialisation and communication with others. Peterson and Siegal (1995) found that deaf children growing up in hearing families experience a significant developmental delay in developing Theory of Mind comparable to that experienced by autistic children. The possible explanation offered for this finding was that deaf children of hearing parents are not able to communicate with others in their environment and share their thoughts, beliefs and feelings as hearing children (or, indeed, deaf children in deaf families) are able to. In a subsequent study, Peterson and Siegal (1997) found that deaf children of deaf parents did not have this developmental delay. Similar results were found by Russell et al. (1998) and in larger scale studies in which language skills were assessed in more detail (deVilliers et al., 2000). Their findings suggest that both the ability to name others' motivations via language, which requires a well-developed vocabulary, and the ability to express one's thoughts about others' motivations, which requires complex syntax, enable children to consider and predict the behaviour of others. This is perhaps not surprising in the light of Luria and Yudovich's assertion that language is important for the consideration of one's *own* motivations and behaviour. Deaf children whose language is impoverished show clear and substantial delays in the development of these conceptual domains.

In this regard, the main problem may be that in the absence of sophisticated (sign) language, communication between non-signing parents and their deaf children remains mainly limited to imperative (i.e. 'do this', 'come there') and first-order intentionality gestures (expressing an awareness of self: 'I am annoyed with you', 'I love you', 'I want you to . . .'). Altruism, guilt and empathy require at least second-order intentionality (an awareness of others' self-awareness), and an appraisal of (the consequences of) how one's behaviour may be interpreted by others requires at least third-order intentionality (an awareness of others' awareness of yourself). In short, second- and third-order intentionality are essential for the ability to display socially appropriate behaviour. Given the aforementioned importance of social norms and values in challenging behaviour, it is easy to see how a lack of second- and third-order intentional thinking is more likely to result in behaviour that is interpreted by others as 'challenging'. Even if such cognitive developmental delays are eventually caught up with, critical stages of psychological development (such as developing intimacy or peer relationships) may already have passed without benefiting from this faculty, and dysfunctional behavioural interaction patterns may have already been established that may be difficult to modify afterwards.

BEHAVIOUR MODIFICATION AND LANGUAGE DELAY

Although many effective behavioural conditioning and reinforcement strategies exist (e.g. Didden *et al.*, 1997), in terms of independent functioning and self-determination in a wide variety of situations, it is desirable that the service user develops conscious insight and choice in his or her behaviour. Consciously deliberated behaviour is more flexible and more likely to be appropriate in novel and diverse settings outside of the relatively narrow situations in which behaviour modification is applied.

Insight can be increased by consistent, concrete and specific feedback of the person's behaviour (which, combined with praise, can be a reinforcement in itself). Such appraisal and feedback mechanisms can be internalised by self-monitoring/recording on concrete criteria (e.g. of how often you exhibited a certain behaviour today) or self-rating/self-evaluation (e.g. observing a video tape of your behaviour and awarding yourself a performance score and reward according to concrete criteria). Internalised feedback facilitates self-reflection, and self-monitoring makes the self-reflective process explicit; they are the basis for the internal dialogue and self-statements that enable self-regulation. A related strategy is 'guided self-talk', which makes explicit the process of internal dialogue and reasoning as the behaviour is performed by saying it out loud to oneself. Harris (1986) points out that poor performance in learning-disabled children is frequently the result of deficits in self-regulation rather than cognitive ability, and that cognitive behaviour modification techniques that emphasise the development of self-regulation through self-statements have been strongly recommended. She examined the natural occurrence of regulatory internal dialogue (or 'private speech') among learning-disabled and normally achieving children during problem-solving, as well as the effects of cognitive behaviour modification training on internal dialogue and task performance. Results certainly indicated significant deficiencies in internal dialogue and task performance among learning-disabled children and that cognitive behaviour modification training resulted in significant improvements. The significance of inner speech in behaviour is also obvious in cognitive behavioural therapy approaches, which encourage a person to examine the role of their 'negative automatic thoughts' (in effect, their internal dialogue) about events in their emotional and behavioural responses to them.

These processes are particularly relevant, but also particularly challenging, when the appropriate language is underdeveloped. Interventions are being developed to promote the emotional development of deaf children (e.g. Hindley *et al.*, 2005) by teaching them an emotional vocabulary and getting them to reflect on their own feelings, those of others and to make a connection between behaviours, how these may be interpreted and their association with feelings. The effectiveness of such interventions is still being evaluated but appears encouraging. How effective such interventions might be for adults, however, who have already passed critical life stages for psychological development and may have firmly entrenched dysfunctional behaviour patterns, is not yet known.

CONCLUSION

In understanding challenging behaviour, it is important to appreciate the perspective of the person exhibiting it, their cognitive faculties, and also that all human behaviour lies on a continuum between instinctual, emotional reaction and conscious, intentional and deliberated action. What allows us to function beyond pure instinct, what sets humans apart from all the other animals and makes us able to do all the things that are astounding, complex and intangibly human, is the level of conscious, rational thought we are able to achieve, and the intentional planned and organised behaviour that is its product. Another is our ability to use language. Moreover, the two go hand in hand. The only way to conceive the abstract is to name it. The only way we can share and achieve a mutual understanding of our complex reasoning, emotion and behaviour is through language. If either cognitive functioning or the ability to use language in thought and communication is disrupted, behaviour is likely to be maladaptive and inappropriate to the circumstances in which it occurs, and more likely to be perceived as 'challenging'. In profound prelingual deafness, there is an increased likelihood that both are the case; as such challenging behaviour in deafness needs to be considered simultaneously from neuropsychological and behavioural, internal-dialogue and functional-communication perspectives (Figure 6.4).

The importance of access to sign language from an early age for profoundly prelingually deaf children is now much more recognised. The establishment of a solid foundation of language, and therefore of cognitive development, is acknowledged as being of priority over (and in fact a prerequisite for) integration in a predominantly hearing world. Whether signed or oral, the crucial issue is that children attain a fully

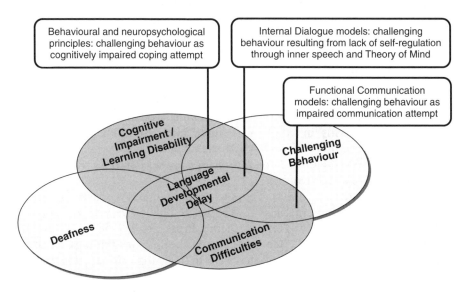

Figure 6.4 Theories and models of challenging behaviours and their relationship to deafness

developed **language**. For centuries, the oral/manual debate has differed on how to achieve this. However, speech does not equal language. Good speech is not a prerequisite for the full development of cognition and adaptive, mature behaviour. Language definitely is.

REFERENCES

Allen D (2000) Recent research on physical aggression in persons with intellectual disability: an overview. *Journal of Intellectual and Developmental Disability* 25(1): 41–58.

Baddeley A (1991) *Human Memory: Theory and Practice*, Hove and London, Lawrence Erlbaum.

Banat D, Summers S, Pring T (2002) An investigation into carers' perceptions of the verbal comprehension ability of adults with severe learning disabilities. *British Journal of Learning Disabilities* 30(2): 7–81.

Benson Yody B, Schaub C, Conway J, Peters S *et al.* (2000) Applied behavior management and acquired brain injury: approaches and assessment. *Journal of Head Trauma Rehabilitation* 15(4): 1041–60.

Berk LE (1992) Children's private speech: an overview of theory and the status of research. In Diaz RM, Berk LE (eds), *Private Speech: From Social Interaction to Self-Regulation*, Hillsdale, NJ, Lawrence Erlbaum, pp. 17–54.

Borthwick-Duffy SA (1994) Prevalence of destructive behaviours. In Thompson T, Gray DB (eds), *Destructive Behaviour in Developmental Disabilities*, Thousand Oaks, CA, SAGE, pp. 3–23.

Braden JP (1992) Intellectual assessment of deaf and hard-of-hearing people: a quantitative and qualitative research synthesis. *School Psychology Review* 21(1): 82–94.

Braden JP (1994) *Deafness, Deprivation and IQ*, New York, Plenum Press.

Bradshaw J (2001) Complexity of staff communication and reported level of understanding skills in adults with intellectual disabilities. *Journal of Intellectual Disability Research* 45(3): 233–43.

Brewin CR (1993) *Cognitive Foundations of Clinical Psychology*, Hove and London, Lawrence Erlbaum.

Carr EG, Durand MV (1994) The social-communicative basis of severe behavioural problems. In Reiss S, Bootzin R (eds), *Theoretical Issues in Behaviour Therapy*, New York, Academic Press, pp. 219–54.

Chamberlain L, Chung MC, Jenner L (1993) Preliminary findings on communication and challenging behaviour in learning. *British Journal of Developmental Disabilities* 39(2): 118–25.

Chung MC, Jenner L, Chamberlain L (1995) One year follow up pilot study on communication skill and challenging behaviour: a pilot study 1. *European Journal of Psychiatry* 9(3): 83–95.

Craig WN, Craig HB (eds) (1993) Tabular summary of schools and classes in the US. *American Annals of the Deaf* 138(2): 169–70.

Crocker S, Edwards L (2004) Deafness and additional difficulties. In Austen S, Crocker S (eds), *Deafness in Mind*, London, Whurr.

Davidson PW, Cain NN, Sloane-Reeves JE, Speybroech AV *et al.* (1994) Characteristics of community-based individuals with intellectual disability and aggressive behavior disorders. *American Journal on Mental Retardation* 98(6): 704–16.

DeVilliers PA, DeVilliers JG, Hoffmeister R, Schick B (2000) Theory of mind development in signing and non-signing Deaf children: the impact of sign language on social-cognition. Paper presented at the 7th International Conference on Theoretical Issues in Sign Language Research, Amsterdam, July 2000.

Didden R, Duker PC, Korzilius H (1997) Meta-analytic study on treatment effectiveness for problem behaviors with individuals who have mental retardation. *American Journal of Mental Retardation* 101(4): 387–99.

Dixon NF (1981) *Preconscious Processes*, Chichester, Wiley.

Emerson E (1995) *Challenging Behaviour: Analysis and Intervention in People with Severe Intellectual Disabilities*, Cambridge, Cambridge University Press.

Hallas C, Fraser W, McGillivary R (1982) *The Care and Training of the Mentally Handicapped*, Edinburgh, Wright.

Harris KR (1986) The effects of cognitive-behavior modification on private speech and task performance during problem solving among learning-disabled and normally achieving children. *Journal of Abnormal Child Psychology* 14(1): 63–76.

Hermelin B, O'Connor N (1964) Crossnodal transfer in normal, subnormal and autistic children. *Neuropsychologia* 2(3): 229–35.

Hindley P, Buxton S, Hussmann C (2005) The emotional development of deaf children at Corner House Inpatient Service. Presentation at the British Society of Mental Health and Deafness Annual Conference, Nottingham, 24 May 2005.

Holt JA (1993) Standard achievement test: 8th edition for deaf and hard of hearing students: reading comprehension subgroup results. *American Annals of the Deaf* 138: 172–5.

Kevan F (2003) Challenging behaviour and communication difficulties. *British Journal of Learning Disabilities* 31: 75–80.

Lazarus RS, Folkman S (1984) *Stress, Appraisal, and Coping*, New York, Springer.

Luria AR (1961) *The role of speech in the regulation of normal and abnormal behavior*, New York, Liveright.

Luria AR, Yudovich FA (1971) *Speech and the Development of Mental Processes in the Child*, London, Penguin.

Mayberry RI (2002) Cognitive development in deaf children: the interface of language and perception in neuropsychology. In Segalowitz SJ, Rapin I (eds), *Handbook of Neuropsychology*, (2nd Edn.), vol. 8, pt. II, pp. 71–107.

McConkey R, Morris I, Purcell M (1999) Communications between staff and adults with intellectual disabilities in naturally occurring settings. *Journal of Intellectual Disability Research* 43(3): 194–205.

Moeller MP (2000) Early intervention and language development in children who are deaf and hard of hearing. *Pediatrics* 106(3): 43–52.

Morris PE (1981) The cognitive psychology of self-reports. In Antaki C (ed), *The Psychology of Ordinary Explanations of Social Behaviour*, London, Academic Press. pp. 185–203.

Norman D, Shallice T (1980) Attention to action: willed and automatic control of behaviour. In Davidson R, Schwartz G, Shapiro D (eds), *Consciousness and self-regulation*, New York, Plenum, vol. 4.

Parkin AJ (1998) The central executive does not exist. *Journal of the International Neuropsychological Society* 4(5): 518–22.

Peterson CC, Siegal M (1995) Deafness, conversation and theory of mind. *Journal of Child Psychology and Psychiatry* 36(3): 459–74.

Peterson CC, Siegal M (1997) Domain specificity and everyday biological, physical, and psychological thinking in normal, autistic, and deaf children. *New Directions for Child Development* 75(Spring): 55–70.

Posner MI, Snyder CR (1975) Attention and cognitive control. In Solso RL (ed), *Information Processing and Cognition: The Loyola Symposium*, Hillsdale, NJ, Lawrence Erlbaum. pp. 55–85.

Russell PA, Hosie JA, Gray CD, Scott C et al. (1998) The development of theory of mind in deaf children. *Journal of Child Psychology and Psychiatry and Allied Disciplines* 39(6): 903–10.

Schroeder SR, Schroeder CS, Smith B, Dalldorf J (1978) Prevalence of self-injurious behaviors in a large state facility for the retarded: a three-year follow-up. *Journal of Autism and Childhood Schizophrenia* 8(3): 261–9.

Shallice T (1988) *From neuropsychology to mental structure*, Cambridge, Cambridge University Press.

Sigafoos J (2000) Communication development and aberrant behaviour in children with developmental disabilities. *Education and Training in Mental Retardation and Developmental Disabilities* 35(2): 168–76.

Skinner BF (1953) *Science and human behavior*, NY, Macmillan.

Stuss DT, Alexander MP (2000) Executive functions and the frontal lobes: a conceptual view. *Psychological Research* 63(3–4): 289–98.

van der Gaag A (1998) Communication skills and adults with learning disabilities: eliminating professional myopia. *British Journal of Learning Disabilities* 26(3): 88–93.

Vygotsky LS (1962) *Thought and language* (trans. Hanfmann E and Vakar G), Cambridge, MA, MIT Press.

Xeniditis K, Russell A, Murphy D (2001) Management of people with challenging behaviour. *Advances in Psychiatric Treatment* 7(2): 109–16.

7

Psychodynamic Approaches to Understanding Challenging Behaviour

CHRISTINE MCPHERSON

> In an institution, the client group can be regarded as the originator of projections with the staff group as the recipients. The staff members may come to represent different, and possibly conflicting, emotional aspects of the psychological state of the client group. (Halton, 1994: 14)

INTRODUCTION

Challenging behaviour can have a disturbing effect on staff working in care settings, undermining their view of themselves as caring and skilled professionals. This chapter will explore the mechanisms through which service users unconsciously attempt to communicate their feelings to staff. It will be argued that often it is only when service users' attempts at communication fail that these feelings are then expressed through openly challenging or aggressive behaviour. Examples will be given to illustrate how unconscious aggression can split the staff team through projection of the service user's conflicts into the staff group. The psychodynamic concepts of **splitting** and **projection** as well as those of **transference** and **countertransference** will be discussed. It will be argued that effective work depends not on staff trying to ignore their disturbed feelings but rather on the ability of staff to allow themselves

Deafness and Challenging Behaviour: The 360° Perspective. Edited by S. Austen and D. Jeffery
© 2007 John Wiley & Sons Ltd

to be disturbed, tolerate their own disturbance and use a reflective stance to understand the information that is being given about the inner world of the service user. It will be suggested that in order to achieve this staff need to be given the opportunity to talk and think about their feelings both individually in supervision and also in supportive staff groups so that appropriate ways of responding can be agreed. Psychodynamic ideas can be applied both within in-patient and other group settings, such as residential, rehabilitation or daycare services. They can also be useful more generally as a way for workers to understand feelings evoked in their work and, therefore, provide more appropriate support to both service users and staff.

EMOTIONAL DEVELOPMENT

Psychodynamic ideas provide a useful way of thinking about unconscious mental processes. This way of thinking about human behaviour can ultimately be traced back to the work of Freud. Freud argued that problems in the present can be a consequence of unresolved emotional difficulties in the past. Storr (1989), writing about the works of Freud, explains Freud's view that the young child, as a way of coping with situations which gave rise to conflicting feelings, learned to repress these feelings (push them down into unconsciousness). **Repression** was seen by Freud as a way of coping or defending against the power of these feelings. However, these repressed feelings did not just disappear but would exert 'powerful pressure' for them to be expressed (Preston-Shoot and Agass, 1990). Freud felt that the individual would then feel quite disturbed and would deploy various defences to enable her/him to return to a state of equilibrium and prevent the repressed feelings from being expressed. It is important to note that in Freud's view defences are essential; everyone uses them and needs them as a way of coping with conflicting feelings. Freud's ideas were developed and modified by later psychoanalysts.

Through her psychoanalytic work with children, Melanie Klein developed the concepts of **splitting** and **projection**; defences which she felt were used to avoid having to experience conflicting feelings towards the same person (Klein, 1946). Klein felt that in early childhood splitting and projection were the predominant defences for avoiding emotional pain. Thus, the conflict between love and hate for the mother, especially when the mother does not provide instant gratification, can be avoided by splitting off the feelings of hate and locating (or **projecting**) them into someone else, maybe a father or a sibling who is at the time getting mother's attention. In normal development, children will slowly learn to tolerate conflicting feelings and realize that they can, for example, have feelings of love and hate/anger towards the same person. In Klein's view, these defences only become pathological when they continue to be used as the child grows up and become the dominant mode of relating to others (Preston-Shoot and Agass, 1990).

Case Study One

Josie, now in her third volatile relationship, wondered why she always found herself with men who became angry and critical of her. She saw herself as a person who was loving and giving and couldn't understand why she felt dissatisfied. With help, she started to own her own angry feelings but also her needy feelings, recognizing that she had always projected them onto others, as a defence against the realization that her early needs for love and attention were not met and her anger about this.

Freud and Klein believed that aggression is an inherited instinct which the individual is able to manage if their instinctual needs for pleasure are gratified. In contrast, Fairbairn (1958) believed that the individual's prime motivation was not pleasure but the need to be in a relationship with an other. For Fairbairn, aggression was 'the result of failure to achieve satisfactory relationships' (de Zulueta, 2003: 108). **Object relations theory** inferred that early relationships with significant others (usually mother or main carer) affect how we relate to others in adult life. The relationships and care we receive in early life become internalized as a psychic or working model. If these early relationships are satisfying, the model we internalize will enable us to make satisfying relationships as we grow up. However, if early experiences are not good, the infant will internalize a model of unsatisfactory relating. In order to protect him/herself from the adverse experiences, the infant's defences will become more rigid and entrenched. The individual might then develop an inner version of reality, built up from their early experiences, which is often an exaggeration of the actual experiences. It will also be mostly unconscious. The individual will then have the expectation that new people they meet will behave in ways similar to the internalized model. Defences will be deployed based on these inner expectations rather than on the current reality. This will make it difficult for them to have a real relationship in the present as the way they see the person they are in relationship with in the present time will be influenced by these inner expectations. Fairbairn calls this a 'closed system of inner reality' (Fairbairn, 1958).

The more difficult the early-life experiences, and the more defences that were built up, the more these defences will be utilized in present relationships. For some people there may be mitigating factors, such as current relationships that temper the adverse affects of early experiences. However, Preston-Shoot and Agass (1990: 31) suggest that 'all individuals to some extent are captives of their own inner worlds'. Those at the healthy end of the spectrum will have fewer expectations of other people and will be more able to see them as they really are. Those at the other end will be so caught up in their own inner version of reality that it will be difficult for them to see people in the present as they really are. For them, 'people are not individuals in their own right and valued as such, but are figures to be coerced into the mould of the inner object' (Sutherland, 1980, p. 847).

Case Study Two

David, a deaf sign language user with a history of mental illness, found it very difficult to engage in a sustained way with people, particularly women, who were trying to support him (e.g. support workers, community nurse). Neglecting his own needs, he would unconsciously coerce those supporting him to think for him and tell him what to do. He would then feel resentful and angry with them. They could not understand what they were doing wrong and assumed it was a feature of his illness. From talking to him and finding out more about his experiences, it became clear that David had experienced his (hearing) mother as overprotective, interfering and disempowering. Staff did not realize that they were reenacting the internalized mother–son relationship with him. By assuming this was a feature of his illness they were unable to understand how his current behaviour related to previous experiences and thus lost an opportunity to forge a stronger therapeutic bond with him.

Bowlby (1979) felt that a secure emotional attachment or 'attunement' between the mother (or significant carer) and the infant were crucial to the infant's ability to develop satisfactory relationships as they grow up and become adults. If early relationships were not satisfactory, later relationships would then be characterized by insecure attachment behaviours. These would take the form of defences, including avoidance of relating, aggression and hostility or ambivalence, all of which would make it difficult for the individual to maintain healthy relationships with others. de Zulueta (2003) cites the work of both Fairbairn (1952) and Bowlby (1984) in arguing that the experience of abuse, early deprivation or failure of attunement make us 'more liable to aggressive or violent behaviour' (de Zulueta, 2003: 183).

The ideas of Winnicott (1954, 1960) and Bion (1959) are also important here. Winnicott felt that the mother's function of 'mirroring', at first through copying the infant's facial expressions and later through putting the child's feelings into words, enables the child to feel 'held' and to develop a secure sense of self. Bion developed the idea of 'containment'. He felt that the young baby is unable to manage or 'contain' their feelings and develops anxiety about them. The baby needs the mother to manage these feelings for them. All being well, the mother will feel the pressure of the baby's feelings of anxiety, which, in psychoanalytic terms, has been 'projected onto' them. The mother will try to understand and 'digest' them and respond in an appropriate way, thus making the baby's anxieties bearable ('containing' them). From this experience, the baby will begin to learn that anxiety as well as other feelings can be managed, will be able to start the process of managing/regulating these for her/himself and will feel confident that help will be available when needed. If these anxieties are not contained, the baby will unconsciously believe that their feelings cannot be managed, will then be unable to regulate them and will unconsciously put pressure on others to manage these feelings as he/she grows up and into adulthood.

EMOTIONAL DEVELOPMENT OF DEAF CHILDREN

Hindley (2000) discusses the early experiences of deaf children and poses the question of whether deaf children are at higher risk of mental health problems. He cites evidence to suggest that a significant minority of deaf children may not have had the early experiences needed to equip them with emotional resilience including the fact that 90% of deaf children are born to hearing parents, the majority of whom do not use sign language. Deaf children are at greater risk of additional impairments, many of which Hindley suggests are well recognized as risk factors for psychiatric disorders. Deaf children are also at higher risk of emotional, physical and sexual abuse than hearing children. Hindley relates how deafness is still often presented as an 'unfortunate sad occurrence' to parents who are often told their aim should be to help their deaf children function as much like hearing children as possible. He cites Koester and Trim's (1991) finding that some hearing mothers appeared to adapt intuitively to their deaf children, but also Gregory *et al.*'s (1995) work, which suggests that a significant minority of hearing parents either never accept their child's deafness or have great difficulty in doing so, with consequent difficulties for their child's view of themselves. Hadadian (1995) discusses studies that found that deaf children's security of attachment was negatively correlated to their parents' attitudes towards deafness. It would seem likely that those parents who did not accept their child's deafness would be less likely to learn alternative communication strategies, such as sign language, to engage with their deaf child. It is difficult to imagine how the mother would be able to help her child contain unmanageable feelings and learn to regulate their own feelings if communication strategies have not been established. However, Hindley (2000) states there is only anecdotal evidence to suggest that poor communication is associated with insecure attachment.

From the above, it would appear that, for a variety of reasons, deaf children are likely to be more emotionally vulnerable than their hearing counterparts and may have difficulties managing their feelings, which can then become manifested in disturbed, often challenging, behaviour. This can continue into adulthood if not resolved by appropriate interventions. Kitson and Thacker (2000) cite Meadow's (1981) research that rates of behaviour disorder in Deaf people are at least twice as common as in hearing people. Linked to the above discussion, it would suggest that a significant proportion of those Deaf people referred to adult mental health services will have had inadequate early experiences of containment and consequent difficulties in managing their feelings.

EMOTIONAL VULNERABILITY AND ITS IMPACT ON STAFF

People who are admitted to in-patient psychiatric settings and many of those in residential units are likely to have had very difficult life experiences and are thus likely to be highly emotionally vulnerable. Hinshelwood (2004: 30) in discussing the extreme emotional vulnerability of those in in-patient psychiatric units suggests that the illness that accounts for their admission 'is something to do with a means of coping with such intolerable feelings'. The patients are, he suggests, vulnerable to and frightened of their own feelings. These feelings can be so intense that often the patient might have difficulty in actually 'being with himself' (Evans, 2005 unpublished paper). Often the patient may be unable to understand or even think about these feelings, possibly through inadequate experiences of containment in early life or due to unresolved feelings related to later trauma. If the person is feeling isolated and insufficiently supported, she or he might use various forms of self-harm as a way of coping with these feelings (Castillo, 2003).

Hinshelwood (2004) believes that patients want staff to understand them and will try different ways of making them understand, often using non-verbal ways as they may have difficulty in understanding and articulating their feelings. If staff still do not understand, the patient will often try more extreme ways of getting them to understand, often through unconscious communication (see below). This can be very disturbing for staff. How staff react will, he feels, influence whether the patient's behaviour escalates or is able to be contained.

Moylan (1994) also discusses unconscious communication, suggesting that in the absence of a common language patients may be driven to use this. She gives an example of a nurse who, when faced with a patient who did not share the same language, felt helpless and unable to use her skills. She also felt impotent and angry that she had to go through this experience and guilty that she was not meeting her usual high standards. In the example given by Moylan, the nurse left the room as soon as she could. It would seem likely that this would be quite a common experience in settings with Deaf service users, particularly for those new to the work. In these settings (residential hostels or in-patient mental health units), the majority of service users will have little or no spoken language and staff will often have limited sign language skills. In the author's experience, many Deaf service users find it difficult to articulate their thoughts and feelings. It is likely therefore that more unconscious communication will be used.

Case Study Three

Robert was admitted to hospital with a psychotic illness. Medication began and he started to improve. However, he then started to refuse medication as well as food. He was detained under the Mental Health Act 1983 so that medication could be administered. However, he continued to refuse food. Staff became angry when discussing Robert and there were often disagreements among the staff group about how to care for him. Staff were unable to come together and acknowledge what was happening and thus lost the opportunity to think about whether these angry feelings might have been unconsciously stirred up by Robert through projection of his angry feelings which he could not allow himself to become aware of. It is possible that anger was never acknowledged in Robert's family and thus he might never have been able to acknowledge and have help with his own angry feelings, unconsciously believing that these were unacceptable. Instead the anger, split off and projected onto members of the staff group, became acted out by them through blaming each other for Robert's deteriorating mental state.

Hinshelwood (2004: 32) suggests that staff should be aware that sometimes 'not getting better' may be 'the expression of some negative emotional state' (the 'negative therapeutic reaction'). The above also illustrates how patients can, through projection, be unconsciously trying to communicate something to us (in this case, anger), which they need help to acknowledge and deal with. In the example of Robert, if we also have difficulty being aware of and managing our own angry feelings, we might unconsciously collude with the patient, lose the opportunity to reflect on our feelings in supervision and risk the staff team being split. Main (1957: 132) writes about the difficulties for staff groups when faced with patients who do not improve with treatment or improve only partially. These patients, he points out, 'had a remarkable capacity to distress those who looked after them'.

Aiyegbusi (2004) suggests that, as professionals, we have our own vulnerabilities, traumas and losses, which may or may not have been processed. Hinshelwood (2004) supports this view that staff are emotionally vulnerable and states that this vulnerability is a common experience for everyone. He writes that if staff find it hard to acknowledge their own anger, for example, they are probably denying their angry feelings, making it very difficult for them to make use of these feelings to gain a better understanding of the service user.

UNCONSCIOUS COMMUNICATION: A RESOURCE FOR STAFF

TRANSFERENCE

The concept of unconscious communication is complex. The concept of **transference** was coined by Freud. Fernando (2004: 78) draws on Bateman and Holmes' (1995) work in describing transference as 'a process that occurs ... when a patient unconsciously transfers onto the therapist feelings previously experienced in relation to significant others'. This links to the previous discussion, where the individual projects their internal reality built up from early experiences in close relationships onto relationships in the present. However, transference does not only occur in therapy. As Preston-Shoot and Agass (1990: 35) point out, 'transference ... describes a phenomenon which is present in some degree in any helping encounter'. Freud at first thought transference was a hindrance to his work, blocking his progress with his patients. However, he later realized it was a powerful tool that could help him to understand his patient's inner world, if he could work with his patient to understand what was being transferred from their past.

Preston-Shoot and Agass (1990) explain that patients may unconsciously put significant pressure on workers to behave in ways they have come to expect from their past experiences, as demonstrated in the previous discussion of David. This pressure could range from obvious attempts at manipulation to quite subtle promptings. Joseph (1985) explains how 'total situations' can be transferred from the past into the present. Staff may not realize that the patient may be unconsciously recreating in the present relationships from their past. If staff can try to understand what is happening, important information can be gained about the patient, information of which the patient themselves may not be consciously aware.

Case Study Four

Susan expected to be let down by her carers, just as she had frequently felt let down by her mother during her childhood. She defended against powerful feelings of rejection and disappointment by frequently missing appointments and thus not allowing herself to become close and have expectations of help from the worker. She was unconsciously transferring onto the worker her internalized expectations from her experiences with her mother. However, in doing this she put pressure on the worker to discharge her and thus risked feeling let down and rejected once again.

COUNTERTRANSFERENCE

Whereas the term 'transference' is used to describe the feelings of the patient or service user in an interaction, the concept of **countertransference** is used to describe the worker's side of the interaction and the feelings evoked in the worker in relation to the service user. To return to the example of Susan:

Case Study Four (revisited)

The worker feels angry and frustrated at being kept waiting when Susan is late or does not turn up at all. She also feels inadequate that she has not been able to engage Susan in the therapeutic process. This results in her feeling very uncomfortable in relation to Susan and she decides to discharge her. However, in doing this the worker is acting out, becoming caught up with Susan in a re-enactment of her early experiences of rejection and disappointment.

The worker's feelings of anger and inadequacy when Susan fails to attend her sessions could prevent her from reflecting on whether she might also be experiencing the projection into her of the split off unwanted feelings of the service user. The difficulty with countertransference feelings is that they can so often become mixed up with our own feelings, particularly when we are not yet fully aware of and comfortable with these feelings ourselves. We may feel uncomfortable, even disturbed, but not sure why. For these feelings to be useful, they need to be thought about carefully and a distinction made between what may be our own feelings from our personal experiences and what may be the patient's feelings projected into us. Money-Kyrle (1956) points out how disturbed the therapist can feel when the patient projects into a part of her or him that has not yet been fully understood. This is why those studying psychodynamic psychotherapy receive their own therapy as part of the training process and regular supervision before and after qualification. It is recognized how easy it can be to get caught up in re-enacting with the patient their early experiences.

The example of Susan shows the importance of trying to understand the service user's behaviour as a re-enactment of early experiences with care givers. If the worker can manage his or her feelings and reflect on them either alone or through supervision or discussion with colleagues together with the information known about Susan, this can provide a valuable means of understanding and thus responding more appropriately to Susan's behaviour, interpreting for her the possible meanings of the missed appointments. If Susan is able to use this information and continue attending, she can be helped to make a start in understanding her inner world, built up from infancy and how this affects her current behaviour.

SUPERVISION AND TRAINING

Staff working in caring settings may feel they have to ignore any feelings they may have towards service users. Aiyegbusi (2004) relates how the trend in psychiatric nursing models has been to avoid thinking about what working with the patient group might be stirring up emotionally. However, Brenman Pick (1985) argues that to make a real therapeutic relationship entails allowing ourselves to be affected at a deep level by the projections of our patients and take time to think about them rather than react so quickly that we avoid experiencing their effect on us. In order to do this, training in psychodynamic concepts as well as regular supervision to provide containment for staff are vital.

Case Study Five

When Brenda (a deaf sign language user) was admitted to the unit, she quickly identified staff she liked and could talk to, showing them her vulnerable side. These staff felt rather special, feeling that only they really understood her. With the other staff (the majority), she was often quite hostile, even aggressive at times. These staff felt that she was manipulative, uncooperative with her care plan and should be discharged as soon as possible. The staff group felt unable to come together to discuss their respective feelings towards Brenda and agree together how to respond to her. Brenda's memories were of parents who were unable to communicate with her and this made it difficult for them to help her to understand and manage her feelings. They were also unable to talk to each other and support each other in managing her feelings and behaviour. Brenda learned to cope with this by manipulating them in an unconscious effort to meet her needs. She felt in control although at the same time she was not having her underlying needs for emotional security and appropriate boundaries met. Brenda was unconsciously re-enacting this scenario in the present with the staff group, putting pressure on them to collude with her in this re-enactment.

The above provides an example of how 'total situations' and ways of relating can be transferred from the past into the present with members of the staff group representing different aspects of Brenda's inner world. Main (1957: 142) describes those very needy patients who cannot manage their own feelings: 'the world would have to manage them because they cannot manage it'. Brenda also provides an example of the type of patient Main discusses who 'divides their world in an attempt to control its imperfections' (Main, 1957: 144) but in doing so also splits the staff team. Main cites Stanton and Schwartz's work (1949a, 1949b, 1949c, 1954) to warn against any 'easy assumptions' that the patient consciously wants to split the team, the patient being 'particularly sensitive to and vulnerable to disharmony in those around them' (Main, 1957: 139). Main agrees with Stanton and Schwartz that 'the patient's distress can be dramatically resolved if the disagreeing staff can meet, disclose and discuss their hidden disagreements and reach genuine consensus about how the patient could be handled in any particular matter' (Main, 1957: 139).

Hinshelwood, writing almost 50 years later, would seem to agree with Main. He discusses the patient who cannot control his feelings and searches for someone to '*be* his self-control' arguing that the patient 'may be as reassured as the staff by effective control of himself' (Hinshelwood, 2004: 30). Hinshelwood appears also to urge caution with the use of the word 'manipulate'. While he agrees that some patients do manipulate our minds (through projection of their feelings into us), he argues that they do this to try to communicate and make us understand their experiences, which through lack of early mirroring and containment they are unable to communicate any other way. When manipulative behaviour occurs, it is often accompanied by splitting of the staff team (as in the example of Brenda above). If staff argue amongst themselves rather than talk together about their different experiences, they may then fail to understand what the patient is trying to communicate. Manipulative behaviour can sometimes be very disturbing for the staff as a group but also as individuals. If the patient feels frightened, for example, they will try to make us understand this feeling by making us feel frightened. Their fear might be of the powerful nature of their own feelings, perhaps fear of their own aggression and not being able to manage it. If we fail to understand this, we may react by becoming defensive. The patient will then feel we have not understood them and will then try in more extreme ways to communicate these feelings so that the worker may feel very disturbed, even under attack. We may then react by refusing to meet the patient alone.

This will merely serve to reinforce to the patient that their feelings are unmanageable. Hinshelwood stresses how important it is for the patient that 'you help her to identify her communicating as distinct from her aggression' (Hinshelwood, 2004: 33).

Hughes and Halek (1991) discuss the benefits of a course in psychodynamic skills, which they feel increased the confidence of in-patient nurses in working therapeutically both with individuals and groups. However, courses in psychodynamic concepts are not generally available in training for mental health professionals. Similarly, Preston-Shoot and Agass, writing for social workers, argue that 'the concepts of transference, countertransference . . . help us to identify certain interpersonal processes which have a crucial bearing, not only on psychotherapy but on all close encounters, especially those of a helping kind' (Preston-Shoot and Agass, 1990: 42). They argue that a working knowledge of psychodynamics should be a basic requirement for all practitioners and 'absolutely essential for supervisors and trainers' (Preston-Shoot and Agass, 1990: 190).

Halton (1994) suggests that the above process, whereby the service user's conflicting emotions are split off and projected into different members of the staff group (as in the example of Brenda above) are inevitable parts of the institutional process. He feels that psychological processes such as splitting and projection, which traditionally have been studied in the mind of the individual, can also happen between individuals or between different parts of an institutional system. He argues that if containment can be offered to the staff group by a consultant, this can help the various parts of the system to become more integrated and thus function more effectively. Obholzer (1994) stresses that for this to happen staff need time together to start the process of understanding each other's roles and perspectives and to eventually develop their own thinking rather than following institutional defensive thinking.

CONCLUSION

This chapter has argued that psychodynamic perspectives can be very useful as ways of thinking about what is happening for service users, trying to understand their inner world but also how this is impacting on their current relationships with professionals. The psychodynamic concepts of splitting, projection, transference and countertransference have been explored to gain an understanding of how these defences can stir up the feelings of staff and affect their ability to forge appropriate therapeutic relationships. Crucially, how staff manage (or 'contain') their own feelings will influence how they respond. It has been argued that deaf service users may have greater difficulties in managing their feelings and thus are likely to be highly dependent on staff to help them to do so. If the unconscious processes can be understood, it is possible that in feeling understood the service users will have less need to act out unbearable feelings as challenging behaviour. It is important that staff are supported and given time to reflect on service users' behaviour and to think about how it may be affecting them as individuals and their work as a staff group. Challenging behaviour can have a powerful negative impact on the work of the staff team, and the psychodynamic approach can offer positive ways to assist the team's therapeutic functioning.

REFERENCES

Aiyegbusi A (2004) Touch and the impact of trauma in therapeutic relationships with adults. In White K (ed), *Touch: Attachment and the Body*, London, Karnac, pp. 49–56.

Bateman A, Holmes J (1995) *Introduction to Psychoanalysis: Contemporary Theory and Practice*, London, Routledge.

Bion W (1959) Attacks on linking. *International Journal of Psychoanalysis* 40: 308–15.

Bowlby J (1979) *The Making and Breaking of Affectional Bonds*, London, Tavistock.

Bowlby J (1984) Violence in the family as a disorder of the attachment and caregiving systems. *The American Journal of Psychoanalysis* 44(1): 9–27.

Brenman Pick I (1985) Working through in the countertransference. *International Journal of Psychoanalysis* 66: 157–66.

Castillo H (2003) *Personality Disorder*, London and Philadelphia, Jessica Kingsley.

de Zulueta F (2003) *From Pain to Violence: The Traumatic Roots of Destructiveness*, London, Whurr.

Evans M (2005) *The Psychoanalytic Supervision of Nurses and Other Mental Health Workers in Psychiatric Settings: Making Room for Madness in Mental Health*, paper presented at the West Midlands Institute for Psychotherapy, 2005.

Fairbairn W (1952) *Psychoanalytic Studies of the Personality*, London, Routledge and Kegan Paul.

Fairbairn W (1958) On the nature and aims of psycho-analytic treatment. *International Journal of Psychoanalysis* 39(5): 374–85.

Fernando J (2004) Psychodynamic considerations in working with people who are deaf. In Austen S, Crocker S (eds), *Deafness in Mind: Working Psychologically with Deaf People Across the Lifespan*, London, Whurr, pp. 75–88.

Gregory S, Bishop J, Sheldon L (1995) *Deaf People and their Families: Developing Understanding*, Cambridge, Cambridge University Press.

Hadadian A (1995) Attitudes towards deafness and security of attachment relationships among young deaf children and their parents. *Early Education and Development* 6(2): 181–91.

Halton W (1994) Some unconscious aspects of organizational life: contributions from psychoanalysis. In Obholzer A, Roberts VZ (eds), *The Unconscious at Work: Individual and Organizational Stress in the Human Services*, London, Routledge, pp. 11–18.

Hindley P (2000) Child and adolescent psychiatry. In Hindley P, Kitson N (eds), *Mental Health and Deafness*, London, Whurr, pp. 42–74.

Hinshelwood RD (2004) *Suffering Insanity: Psychoanalytic Essays on Insanity*, Hove and New York, Brunner-Routledge.

Hughes PM, Halek C (1991) Training nurses in psychotherapeutic skills. *Psychoanalytic Psychotherapy* 5(2): 115–23.

Joseph B (1985) Transference: the total situation. In Feldman M, Bott Spillius E (eds), *Psychic Equilibrium and Psychic Change*, London, Routledge, pp. 156–67.

Kitson N, Thacker A (2000) Adult psychiatry. In Hindley P, Kitson N (eds), *Mental Health and Deafness*, London, Whurr, pp. 74–98.

Klein M (1946) Notes on some schizoid mechanisms. *International Journal of Psycho-Analysis* 33: 433–8.

Koester LS, Trim VM (1991) *Face-to-face Interactions With Deaf and Hearing Infants: Do Maternal or Infant Behaviours Differ?* Paper presented at the Biennial Meeting of the Society of Research in Child Development. Seattle, USA, 18–20 April 1991.

Main T (1957) The ailment. *British Journal of Medical Psychology* 30(3): 129–45.

Meadow KP (1981) Studies of the behaviour problems of deaf children. In Stein L, Mindel E, Jabaley T (eds), *Deafness and Mental Health*, New York, Grune & Stratton, pp. 3–22.

Money-Kyrle RE (1956) Normal countertransference and some of its deviations. *International Journal of Psychoanalysis* 37(4–5): 360–6.

Moylan D (1994) The dangers of contagion: projective identification processes in institutions. In Obholzer A, Roberts VZ (eds), *The Unconscious at Work: Individual and Organizational Stress in the Human Services*, London, Routledge, pp. 51–9.

Obholzer A (1994) Fragmentation and integration in a school for physically handicapped children. Obholzer A, Roberts VZ (eds), *The Unconscious at Work: Individual and Organizational Stress in the Human Services*, London, Routledge, pp. 84–93.

Preston-Shoot M, Agass D (1990) *Making Sense of Social Work: Psychodynamics, Systems and Practice*, Basingstoke and New York, Palgrave Macmillan.

Stanton AH, Schwartz MS (1949a) The management of a type of institutional participation in mental illness. *Psychiatry* 12: 13–26.

Stanton AH, Schwartz MS (1949b) Medical opinion and the social context in the mental hospital. *Psychiatry* 12: 243–9.

Stanton AH, Schwartz MS (1949c) Observations on dissociation as social participation. *Psychiatry* 12: 339–54.

Stanton AH, Schwartz MS (1954) *The Mental Hospital*, New York, Basic Books.

Storr A (1989) *Freud*, Oxford, Oxford University Press.

Sutherland J (1980) The British object relations theorists: Balint, Winnicott, Faribairn, Guntrip. *Journal of American Psychoanalytic Association* 28(4): 829–60.

Winnicott D (1954) Metapsychological and clinical aspects of regression within the Psycho-analytical set-up. In Winnicott D (ed), (1958) *Collected Papers: Through Pediatrics to Psychoanalysis*, London, Hogarth, pp. 278–94.

Winnicott D (1960) The Theory of the Parent–Infant Relationship. In Winnicott D (1965), *The Maturational Processes and the Facilitating Environment*, London, Karnac, pp, 37–55.

8

Autistic Spectrum Disorder, Deafness and Challenging Behaviour

PAT COLLINS AND STEVE CARNEY

INTRODUCTION

This chapter addresses the issues of a group of conditions covered by the term 'Autistic Spectrum Disorder' and how this may present in Deaf sign language users. There is little formal research in this area and even less when we come to address how challenging behaviour can develop and be managed. We will also consider the implications of co-morbidity for this group, the difficulties in diagnosis, the problems of accessing appropriate services and recommendations to aid management.

WHAT IS AUTISTIC SPECTRUM DISORDER?

Since cases were first described by Kanner (1943), there has been considerable debate as to whether there are distinct disorders within Autistic Spectrum Disorder (ASD) or whether there is merely a continuum with the same features present in differing degrees.

While there remains different emphasis on the importance of certain features in the subgroups, there is broad agreement on the criteria to be met internationally as shown in the *International Classification of*

Deafness and Challenging Behaviour: The 360° Perspective. Edited by S. Austen and D. Jeffery
© 2007 John Wiley & Sons Ltd

Diseases (ICD-10, World Health Organization, 1992) and *Diagnostic and Statistical Manual of Mental Disorders* (DSM-IV) (American Psychiatric Association, 1994).

A diagnosis of autism (F84.0) requires the following features:

> A type of pervasive developmental disorder that is defined by: (a) the presence of abnormal or impaired development that is manifest before the age of three years, and (b) the characteristic type of abnormal functioning in all the three areas of psychopathology: reciprocal social interaction, communication, and restricted, stereotyped, repetitive behaviour. In addition to these specific diagnostic features, a range of other non-specific problems are common, such as phobias, sleeping and eating disturbances, temper tantrums, and (self-directed) aggression. (WHO, 1992, p. 275)

The criteria for Asperger's syndrome (F84.5) are as follows:

> A disorder of uncertain nosological validity, characterized by the same type of qualitative abnormalities of reciprocal social interaction that typify autism, together with a restricted, stereotyped, repetitive repertoire of interests and activities. It differs from autism primarily in the fact that there is no general delay or retardation in language or in cognitive development. This disorder is often associated with marked clumsiness. There is a strong tendency for the abnormalities to persist into adolescence and adult life. Psychotic episodes occasionally occur in early adult life. (WHO, 1992, p. 286)

HOW DOES ASD PRESENT IN DEAF PEOPLE?

Broadly speaking, ASD presents in much the same way in Deaf people as in those who are hearing. Communication differences in ASD can be blatant or subtle. For Deaf people with ASD, it is therefore important to involve staff and carers who are skilled in sign language. Deaf staff especially can point out what are often subtle differences in communication. There will be differences in grammar, pronoun reversal, pedantic and repetitive signing as for those who use speech. Signing can be disrupted by motor coordination problems causing errors that may not be regarded as important by the person with ASD. They may avoid eye contact, which not only prevents them understanding what is said to them but also reduces the amount of information that can be given to the observer.

Many of these difficulties are heightened by an associated deficiency in Theory of Mind. This theory was first presented by Premack and Woodruff (1978) and is the ability to appreciate that others can hold their own beliefs, desires and intentions which may be different and separate from one's own. It seems possible from this that a lack of empathy and poor ability to engage wholeheartedly in communication would follow if Theory of Mind were impaired. Indeed, many studies have shown that this is so (Baron-Cohen *et al.*, 1985, 1986; Perner *et al.*, 1989; Reed and Peterson, 1990; Swettenham *et al.*, 1996). Consequently, the individual with communication difficulties, such as those noted above, does not consider them a problem and does not correct them. Nor does he or she make allowances for those having difficulty understanding them. Indeed, it is not uncommon for people with ASD to become frustrated with those who fail to understand them.

PREVALENCE OF ASD

Autistic Spectrum Disorder is found through all demographic groupings and affects as many as 1 in 110 people (Barnard *et al.*, 2001). In 1995, Wolff estimated a prevalence of 71 per 10 000 (Wolff, 1995). For autism alone, the prevalence is much lower but still varies widely. Early studies based on Kanner's original criteria found as few as 4.5 per 10 000 affected (Lotter, 1966); later work gives figures as much as ten times this (Wing and Gould, 1979; Ehlers and Gillberg, 1993).

Given that prevalence results differ so widely in hearing people, it is difficult to draw comparisons between the hearing and Deaf communities. One study found that in a group of children with hearing impairment 5.3% met criteria for autism (Jure *et al.*, 1991). However, since many of the suggested causes of autism are also associated with deafness, it would not be surprising to see a higher prevalence of ASD within the Deaf population than in the general population.

PREVALENCE OF CHALLENGING BEHAVIOUR IN PEOPLE WITH ASD

Challenging behaviour can include aggression, self-harm, destructive acts, resistance and so on. Depending on the context and the severity, it is usually managed within the home, education or mental health

service in which is occurs. Occasionally, however, challenging behaviour falls within the jurisdiction of the criminal justice system.
Ghaziuddin *et al.*(1991) looked at reports of 132 people with Asperger's
syndrome in the US and found that only three had a clear history of
violent behaviour. They conclude that this is much lower than the 7%
of 20 to 24-year-olds involved in violent crime in the US.

Unfortunately, in the author's experience, mild to moderate episodes
of challenging or criminal behaviour in people with ASD (and in Deaf
people) often go unrecorded as many within the criminal justice system
feel sorry for them, are then overly lenient and do not proceed with
any legal action other than a ride home in a police car. This can then
further reinforce the behaviour.

Wing (1997) lists reasons for offending behaviour in those with
ASD

- pursuit of special interest
- experiences of bullying and rejection and desire for revenge
- hostility towards a family member and blame
- oversensitivity to incoming stimuli leading to high arousal and violent
  behaviour, either towards the stimulus or at random
- passively following the lead of a stronger personality
- a cry for help
- lack of awareness of wrongdoing
- a purely intellectual interest in the crime detaching from the emotional effects of the victim.

In 1999, Hare *et al.* were commissioned to establish the incidence of
ASD in those detained under the Mental Health Act 1983 in English
secure hospitals. They found only a small portion of those within
special hospitals had ASD. They found that the statistics for homicide
and violent crime within the ASD group were comparable for the total
population. They have a lower incidence of sex crime but a higher one
for arson. There has been no estimate of the number of Deaf people
with ASD in prison.

DIAGNOSTIC DIFFICULTIES

Differential diagnosis involving ASD is often problematic. ASD mimics
many other psychiatric conditions and, when accompanied by certain
features of developmental deprivation, deafness mimics ASD.

ASD as a condition falls between many stools: learning disability, social care, mental health services and often the person with ASD has been passed between numerous services, each claiming not to have the appropriate expertise. Few clinicians have experience of working with people with ASD and even fewer with Deaf people who have ASD. Those deciding upon service provision for Deaf people with ASD may have debated which expertise the client can best tolerate being absent: would they be better treated by the service that has limited knowledge of deafness or the service that has limited knowledge of ASD? Co-working and close liaison is, of course, the solution.

Out-patient assessment may be sufficient to diagnose ASD. However, Deaf services tend to cover large catchment areas such that thorough out-patient assessment is unrealistic and in-patient assessment often necessary. In cases of challenging behaviour, it may seem more appropriate to remove the patient from the home environment. However, for clients with ASD the change of venue is likely to exacerbate their anxiety and enhance the symptomatology, possibly increasing physical risk to the patient, staff and others. Being away from carers who know the person well may result in misunderstanding and mismanagement of the individual.

A detailed history both from the carer and general nursing observations is vital in order to make a correct diagnosis. Within Deaf services, a native signer is ideally included in the assessment as a relay interpreter to aid communication and to ensure that normal communication styles for Deaf people are not misinterpreted as indicating signs of ASD.

DEAFNESS MIMICKING ASD

When considering developmental history, one needs to bear in mind the limited access a Deaf child has to children of their own age due to cultural, social and language barriers. Similarly, discord in the culture, language and the family relationship at home can produce adverse effects by limiting social experiences and opportunities for shared learning. This may lead to impaired social skills and limited relationships in future years. Parents' reports of schooling are often sketchy and unclear if the child moves away to residential school and parents rely on brief school reports.

Historically, hearing parents of Deaf children were strongly discouraged to sign with their child but to encourage their use of speech, to enable them to fit into the hearing world. Schools also prohibited signing and emphasised learning speech at the expense of academic achievement and learning social norms and values (Austen and Coleman, 2004). Without a common language and the ability to express themselves, the Deaf child grows up linguistically, emotionally and socially isolated. The child is unable to pick up on social cues from family members, and general information is unavailable to them unless they are informed directly. General discussions and debates that hearing individuals can learn from, for example from background radio, TV and newspapers, are not accessible. Even where a child and/or family do sign, there may be few others in the locality with whom to communicate and a child may grow up relatively isolated.

The result of this deprivation may be a presentation that mimics ASD.

- concrete thinking, lack of empathy, poor theory of mind
- limited socialisation and abnormal social development
- abnormal behaviour.

All Deaf mental health services receive numerous referrals regarding individuals who have experienced deprivation and who appear to have ASD. Often, one of the most effective diagnostic tools is to provide the Deaf person with increased peer contact and sign language over a prolonged period to see if symptoms reduce. In the absence of ASD, certain behaviours, such as the need for routine, will reduce.

However, some of the effects of deprivation will persist. Where such Deaf people have eventually acquired their cultural language through college and social circles, such as local Deaf clubs and organised events, they still have difficulties with cognitive impairment (concrete thinking and poor Theory of Mind) and psychological difficulties due to the lack of language in their formative years.

Writers in the early 1960s did not recognise deprivation and concluded that this presentation was characteristic of Deaf people in general. Basilier (1964) applies the term 'surdophrenia' or 'deaf mind' to this description. Later, this was refined to explain that any of these features were related to being immersed in Deaf culture (Altshuler, 1971; Misiaszek *et al.*, 1985). These views have now fallen out of favour as they are felt to be pejorative and unhelpful (Swaans-Joha, 1991).

An awareness of Deaf culture is crucial to be able to differentially diagnose ASD in Deaf people. While some Deaf people use excessive detail and repetition in their discourse, which can represent an autistic fascination with detail or inability to assess what the 'listener' needs to know, this same detail and repetition can be a feature of normal story-telling in Deaf culture.

Ainsworth *et al.* (1978) report that Deaf children's relationships with their hearing mothers often demonstrate insecure attachment. This may be because problematic communication prevents the formation of the crucial bond, normally formed when people have a common language, and the family are not able to offer the infant the security and reassurances necessary to establish an integrated personality. This can result in the parent becoming anxious in their interactions with the child or even distancing from the child, who subsequently forms an anxiety attachment and has problems in learning to trust their surroundings and relationships with others. This can then present as abnormal social development and behaviour, which can mimic aspects of ASD.

ASD MIMICKING OTHER PSYCHIATRIC DIAGNOSES

Schizophrenia, ASD and Deafness

For the person with ASD the tendency for limited facial expression, reduction in spontaneous movements, paucity of expressive gestures, affective non-responsiveness, lack of vocal inflection, affective flattening and latency of response can all lead to a misdiagnosis of schizophrenia. The crucial differentiating feature is time of onset. These symptoms presenting as a recent change in the individual's behaviour would be seen in a history of schizophrenia, whereas this presentation as a premorbid state points to ASD. The individual may also have slow and tangential responses to questions and shortened responses in order to reduce awkwardness, which adds to the difficulty of assessment.

The tendency for a person with ASD to have concrete thinking and limited ability to understand how others think may result in the person being labelled as paranoid; misinterpreting social contact can also lead to inappropriate emotional responses contributing to this impression. People with ASD are at no more risk of developing schizophrenia than the general population (Volkmar and Cohen, 1991). Long-standing discussions about schizoid personality in people with ASD and the propensity to develop into schizophrenia are refuted by many, including Tantum (2000).

Case Study One

Mr S is a 24-year-old Deaf man who was admitted for assessment due to increasing violence towards his parents, with whom he lived. He was diagnosed with a schizophreniform illness and ASD. He returned home and was settled though he had 'negative symptoms' and loss of usual interests. After two years, his mother gave up work and began to look after her own increasingly frail mother, requiring her to spend nights away from Mr S. Mr S grew steadily more anxious and started signing to himself. His medication increased, to which he objected and became agitated. He ultimately made a prolonged assault on his mother and was detained for assessment. He settled quickly having been familiar with the environment and signing staff. No further psychotic symptoms were observed and it was concluded that this was a stress reaction, related to his ASD, due to the environmental changes at home.

Obsessive-compulsive Disorder, ASD and Deafness

As a result of the enduring rituals and routines that someone with ASD uses to maintain a sense of order and predictability, there is often a rush to diagnose obsessive-compulsive disorder (OCD). A clear history is necessary to identify whether these symptoms have been present since early childhood (ASD) or of more recent onset (OCD). In OCD, the individual maintains their social or emotional reciprocity and empathy, which would not be seen in ASD. OCD in Deaf people presents in much the same way as in hearing people.

Ghaziuddin *et al.* (1992) differentiate the stereotyped behaviours from those found in OCD, in that there is no subjective report of distress and compulsion to perform. Fitzgerald and Corvin (2001) feel that the rituals and obsessive interests are not experienced as ego-dystonic but are often enjoyed, compared to the persistent intrusive thoughts and impulses of the person with OCD, which often relate to some belief that the obsessional behaviours will avert a catastrophic event or reduce stress.

Depression and Affective Disorders, ASD and Deafness

People with ASD are more susceptible to affective disorders, owing to the confusing nature of their surroundings and the resulting anxiety.

Although research shows there is no more co-morbidity of other clinical conditions in ASD than the general population, there is a higher incidence of depression, anxiety disorders and bipolar disorder (Gillberg and Billstedt, 2000). Depression is often the result of loss, and for someone with ASD the concept of loss is far less tangible than for others. An episode can be triggered by such things as a slight change in routine or the loss of an object.

There are difficulties in diagnosing depression for this group. Owing to a poverty of content of speech, concrete ways of describing physical and emotional experiences, the individual may not be able to describe their feelings so much as show them in altered behaviour, which could in some cases be challenging. Similarly, in Deaf individuals who have had impoverished linguistic development it may also be difficult to recognise affective disorder. Limited language to describe feelings and inexperience of medical terms will mean that the clinician will need to use more descriptive signs to establish feelings, emotions and experiences.

The individual's set routines may make it difficult for the observer or carer to notice any changes in their affect or behaviour. Indeed, if a carer notices a change in routine they may just attribute it to 'a phase'. Alongside the difficulties in expressing distress and emotions, this may result in a long delay in diagnosis and result in the eventual presentation being quite severe.

Mania, ASD and Deafness

Many of the symptoms of ASD – for example excessive talk (particularly regarding specialist interests), distractibility, sleep problems (namely reduced sleep or altered patterns), lack of fear of danger, irritability, overactivity, social disinhibition and changes in affect in response to change and other situations – can easily be misdiagnosed as mania. Hypomania can be confused with the individual's everyday way of excitable conversation or talk about their fantastic, grandiose, imaginary ideas or preoccupations.

Case Study Two

A young Deaf man was admitted for assessment following an allegation of rape made against him. His own views on the incident did not seem compatible with the evidence. He also had overvalued ideas of building a business and had gained numerous bank loans to do this. He had some understanding of finances but had no qualifications or experience in business. There was much debate as to whether this was a case of grandiose ideas with hypomania or simply overvalued ideas as in Asperger's syndrome. He was unable to see the harm he had caused by either the rape or the bank loans, but the court cases were ultimately dropped. From further inquiries, it eventually transpired that he had always been a loner at school unless talking enthusiastically and repeatedly about his plans to build a business and had never had a sexual relationship.

The person with ASD who actually becomes manic may show changes such as increased or unusual agitation, non-compliance with ordinary routines and expectations, destructiveness, lack of sleep, increased hyperactivity, increased interest activity, increase in repetitive behaviours and pleasure-seeking activities. Lainhart (1999) sees this as a worsening of baseline features. Ironically, mood changes to signify both depression and mania are not always clearly seen but can present similarly with a change in behaviour, usually in increased activity and irritability. It is therefore important to check mood changes against environmental changes and stresses. Once again, the additional communication difficulties need to be remembered by clinicians when assessing Deaf people in these circumstances.

MANAGING CHALLENGING BEHAVIOUR IN DEAF PEOPLE WITH ASD

Where Deaf clients with ASD present to services it may be that their challenging behaviour is associated with either the deafness, the ASD or with a co-morbid condition such as schizophrenia or depression. When diagnosis is delayed, there is an increased risk of maladaptive coping strategies being adopted and new behaviours developing. So even after the presenting condition has been diagnosed and treated the behaviour can continue.

Challenging behaviour in Deaf people with ASD is the same behaviour as presented by anyone else. Modifying or preventing the behaviour, however, may need different methods and understanding, with particular emphasis on communication issues. It is difficult for individuals with ASD to maintain eye contact with others. This can lead to errors in communication, which can produce frustration and possibly behavioural problems. It might be difficult for staff and carers to understand why the service user is distressed or angry. Furthermore, it might then be even more difficult to engage the individual when they are refusing eye contact.

It is vital that staff and carers are well acquainted with the client's normal patterns of behaviour and to avoid outbursts by building up details of likely triggers. It is worth remembering that there may be a considerable time lag between a trigger and any challenging behaviour, which means that it is often difficult to make the link.

ENVIRONMENT

In providing services to people who are Deaf and have ASD, environment plays a huge part in their comfort. Individuals who prefer and function better with their own personal space will benefit from environments with small groups of people and purpose-designed rooms. Attention to communication is imperative. Staff need to have adequate signing skills, Deaf awareness and be aware of the need for total communication.

The need for predictability, routine and structure is pivotal to managing anxiety and subsequent problem behaviours for the person with ASD. Any intervention needs to be carried out in each of his or her varying environments (home, school, college, work etc.), as people with ASD find it hard to generalise from one situation to another. In order to manage this on an acute in-patient psychiatric ward (Deaf or hearing), there will always be difficulties regarding continuity due to factors such as the unpredictable nature of the mental health status of the other patients, staff duty rotas and presence of temporary staff.

ROUTINES AND RITUALS

An area that often causes difficulties for services is rituals and obsessive behaviour. The rituals themselves can be challenging by causing time-keeping problems, distress to others or harm to the individual. Interruption of the ritual is likely to cause anxiety and potentially challenging behaviour as a response.

For the person with ASD, the routine helps to reduce any anxiety produced from the poor understanding of their environment and from not knowing what is expected of them from even an hour-to-hour basis.

When admitted to either a generic or Deaf ward for assessment, the individual may not be able to carry out these routines owing to limitations of the environment and consideration of other service users. This can result in an escalation of behaviour, which the clinician needs to address in a sympathetic manner, understanding that it is related to anxiety and the need for sameness, and not through more negative attributes.

CONSISTENCY AND PLANNING

The often prolonged periods of anxiety-driven behaviour can exhaust clinicians whose responses may change depending on their own mental or emotional state. This lack of continuity or consistency can act as a further stimulation for anxiety and have a detrimental effect on challenging behaviour.

Case Study Three

Mr X, a Deaf man with ASD, was referred to the team due to isolative behaviour and a loss of his special interests. He had poorly controlled epilepsy and generalised anxiety. He would often have anger outbursts towards his elderly parents. It became apparent he was concerned about having a seizure while out of the home and so a desensitisation programme was initiated. This started from the signing environment of a specialist Deaf mental health in-patient ward and then gradually extended to shopping expeditions, which he seemed to enjoy. He developed a relationship with the worker and knew what was expected of him, and his anxiety reduced from the predictability of the weekly event. Unfortunately, when the worker was no longer able to provide the time needed and replaced by another person, Mr X reverted back to his formal behaviours with even more severity, refusing to go out even with his parents as he had done so before. This identifies the need for consistency and planning for change in managing maladaptive coping behaviours.

APPROPRIATE REINFORCEMENT

People with disabilities or differences are often considered less capable of being responsible for their own actions. It can be challenging and time-consuming to make a Deaf person with ASD aware which behaviours are acceptable, unacceptable and criminal. As a result, some will receive inappropriate reinforcement. Just as the criminal justice system shows misplaced sympathy or avoids time-consuming and frustrating interventions, so might clinicians and educators. In the absence of consistent rewarding of appropriate behaviour and extinguishing of inappropriate behaviour, challenging behaviour will continue.

Where the behaviour extends to the criminal, most professionals would advise that Deaf offenders, including those with ASD, should be brought within the normal legal framework (so long as they are granted as full access as possible by means of qualified, experienced interpreters and Deaf relay interpreters).

TOUCHING PEOPLE WITH ASD

Touching, for example to get a Deaf person's attention, is a normal part of Deaf culture. Many people with ASD will abhor physical contact, particularly when it is unexpected. At times of escalating behaviour, rather than encouraging the individual to stop being aggressive, it may induce a severe fight-or-flight reaction. When intervening in challenging behaviour, de-escalation is always preferable to restraint and particularly so when the individual has ASD. It is crucial that staff have training in both sign language and ASD. For staff that have less than adequate signing and a poor understanding of sensory overload, their efforts to guide or restrain a Deaf person with ASD may be counterproductive.

COMMUNICATION

Communication is an obvious issue when clients are deaf, but communication difficulties are also a primary part of ASD. It is important to recognise that people with ASD may not be able to tolerate extensive contact with the patient. Achieving this balance between being available and encouraging communication and giving the person space can be extraordinarily difficult.

Case Study Four

During his second in-patient admission, Mr S began waiting outside the kitchen, pressing the access code. His communication was minimal with delayed responses; so when staff asked what he wanted he did not reply. This continued for two days until he was curtly told by staff to stop. He became frustrated and kicked the door resulting in his having to visit the Accident and Emergency department. His community nurse, who knew him well, asked about this. He signed 'chocolate milk'. The nurse took him into the kitchen where upon Mr S opened the fridge and there indeed was his chocolate milk. Poor understanding of the communication needs of people with ASD is often the cause of management issues and should be minimised during an assessment.

Teachh

The Treatment and Education of Autistic and Related Communication Handicapped Children (Schopler, 1994) is a flexible supplementary communication system enabling the individual to increase independence while lessening anxiety states. It uses a visual display board of the activities in which the individual is expected to partake using photographs or simple Makaton or widget symbols (Detheridge and Detheridge, 2002). The individual is encouraged to set up the board for the allotted time and refers to it prior to each activity to learn the expected routine and to reduce uncertainty and anxiety. Although the use of such communication boards with Deaf people has not been documented, the additional communication information within the pictures and symbols should add extra understanding and independence for Deaf people with ASD.

Social Stories

These are short stories that are aimed at people with ASD to help them understand their social world and behave 'appropriately' within it. They are specific and unambiguous, avoiding metaphors, which those with ASD have difficulty understanding. They provide important clues and responses, thus avoiding the individual's need to make assumptions (Gray, 2000). They can be used alongside social training activities and be most beneficial within new environments, such as the in-patient unit. Again, there have been no studies of their use with Deaf individuals but should be easily incorporated into their management plan.

Picture Exchange Communication System (PECS)

These are visual ways to augment communication to help the individual with the spoken word (Bondy and Frost, 1994) or help the Deaf person with sign. The level of visual interpretation and integration needs assessing so a more simplistic symbol line drawing may be easier to understand. Sometimes words accompany the picture, as the written word is easier for the person with ASD to understand than the spoken word. With a Deaf person's varied academic ability, this may help or hinder. PECS is a graduated system that encourages the person to identify, learn and make choices and engage in two-way communication.

HOUSING PROVISION

Carers are still the main source of support for the individual with ASD. Barnard *et al.* (2001) highlight the need for local health and social services to develop services together, addressing issues of education, housing and employment for the hearing population. Nationally, for Deaf people there are very few care homes for those with mental health problems. There are hardly any that are structured specifically to care for Deaf people with ASD. There is nearly always some compromise made regarding either the level of the signing environment or the level of expertise of staff in managing problems of ASD. Often these patients are placed in care homes for Deaf people with mental health problems. They are small homes, as described above, but obviously they do not meet the needs of Deaf people who have ASD or similar traits that are ready to move on from living with parents or have had sufficient mental health problems that their families and carers can no longer cope.

Case Study Five

Miss T was a young woman who had been placed in a care home for Deaf people after the death of her mother. She had not previously been in contact with mental health services but had been assessed as being unable to be supported at home alone. Within one week she had assaulted a Deaf member of staff, damaged the door to the office and ran off on two occasions and needed returning by the police. Further investigation revealed that her mother hardly used any formal sign language and they mostly used mime and some signs they developed together. The environment was Deaf-friendly and fully signing but was overwhelming for her. At home she was used to having free access at all times to all rooms in the house. The only time this was denied was when her mother was dying and her family kept her mother's room closed. The office door was often closed for meetings, possibly invoking anxiety related to her mother's death.

Where housing away from the parental home is indicated, Deaf people with ASD are often shunted between services and accommodation for those with a learning disability and psychiatric services in an effort to find somewhere they can settle. This is usually done by having a number of visits to different care homes leading to an overnight stay for increasing periods. While this is well intended, people with ASD are often destabilised by this and find the idea of making choices very difficult. It is not uncommon to find that attempts at resettlement fail during the trial period or shortly after.

Sometimes it can be appropriate for individuals to be placed with specialist services for hearing people with ASD. In view of the often limited and idiosyncratic communication styles, it can be easier to provide communication support to such a service and then using the expertise of staff skilled in dealing with the problems of the underlying disorder. Reducing the sensory input by being removed from a Deaf environment allows some patients to flourish.

CONCLUSION

Autistic Spectrum Disorders are often difficult to diagnose and manage. This is equally true in the Deaf and hearing populations. As communication difficulty is a prominent feature, the added complication of deafness and the need to use the individual's own language can make for even greater difficulties. It is essential that those working in this field have the appropriate skills and knowledge of sign language and Deaf awareness. Failure to do so will more likely result in misunderstanding and greater levels of challenging behaviour.

It is important to consider other diagnoses which can complicate the picture and trigger difficult behaviour, but it is equally important to be aware of factors in the environment and internal world of the Deaf person with ASD that can produce problems. Knowledge of the individual's routines and patterns of behaviour is crucial to being able to resolve such difficulties.

Currently, there are very few resources to help Deaf people with ASD. When challenging behaviour presents, the acute mental health services are ill equipped to cope and there are few mental health services specifically for Deaf people. Even here there are limited resources and expertise. Good-quality residential care for people with ASD is difficult to find and it is even harder to locate any placements that can meet the needs of Deaf residents. As a result, such individuals are often placed in less appropriate homes for hearing people or in Deaf environments with limited experience of managing the problems of ASD.

REFERENCES

Ainsworth MDS, Blehart MC, Waters E, Wall S (1978) *Patterns of Attachment: A Physiological Study of the Strange Situation*, Hillsdale, NJ, Lawrence Erlbaum.

Altshuler K (1971) Studies of the deaf: relevance to psychiatric theory. *American Journal of Psychiatry* 12711: 1521–6.

American Psychiatric Association (1994) *Diagnostic and Statistical Manual of Mental Disorders*, Washington, American Psychiatric Association.

Austen S, Coleman E (2004) Controversy in deafness: *Animal Farm* meets *Brave New World*. In Austen S, Crocker S (eds), *Deafness in Mind: Working Psychologically with Deaf People Across the Lifespan*, London, Whurr, pp. 3–20.

Barnard J, Harvey V, Potter D, Prior A (2001) *Ignored or Ineligible: The Reality for Adults with Autistic Spectrum Disorders*, London, National Autistic Society.

Baron-Cohen S, Leslie AM, Frith U (1985) Does the autistic child have a 'Theory of mind'? *Cognition* 211: 37–46.

Baron-Cohen S, Leslie AM, Frith U (1986) Mechanical, behavioural and intentional understanding of picture stories in autistic children. *British Journal of Developmental Psychology* 4: 113–25.

Basilier T (1964) Surdophrenia. The psychic consequences of congenital or early acquired deafness. Some theoretical and clinical considerations. *Acta Psychiatrica Scandinavica* 40(suppl. 180): 363–72.

Bondy A, Frost L (1994) The Picture Exchange Communication System. *Focus on Autistic Behaviour* 9(3): 1–19.

Detheridge T, Detheridge M (2002) *Literacy Through Symbols: Improving Access for Children and Adults*, London, David Fulton.

Ehlers S, Gillberg C (1993) The epidemiology of Asperger syndrome: a total population study. *Journal of Child Psychology and Psychiatry* 34(8): 1327–50.

Fitzgerald M, Corvin A (2001) Diagnosis and differential diagnosis of Asperger syndrome. *Advances in Psychiatric Treatment* 7(4): 310–8.

Ghaziuddin M, Tsai LY, Ghaziuddin N (1991) Brief report: violence in Asperger syndrome, a critique. *Journal of Autism and Developmental Disorders* 21(3): 349–54.

Ghaziuddin M, Tsai LY, Ghaziuddin N (1992) Co-morbidity of autistic disorder in children and adolescents. *European Child and Adolescent Psychiatry* 1(4): 209–13.

Gillberg C, Billstedt E (2000) Autism and Asperger's syndrome: co-existence with other clinical disorders. *Acta Psychiatrica Scandinavica* 102(5): 321–30.

Gray AC (2000) *The New Social Stories Book*, Texas, Future Horizons.

Hare DJ, Gould J, Mills R, Wing L (1999) *A Preliminary Study of Individuals with Autistic Spectrum Disorder in Three Special Hospitals in England*, Bromley, National Autistic Society.

Jure R, Rapin I, Tuchman RF (1991) Hearing-impaired autistic children. *Developmental Medicine and Child Neurology* 33(12): 1062–72.

Kanner L (1943) Autistic disturbances of affective contact. *Nervous Child* 2: 217–50.

Lainhart JE (1999) Psychiatric problems in individuals with autism, their parents and siblings. *International Review of Psychiatry* 11(4): 278–98.

Lotter V (1966) Epidemiology of autistic conditions in young children I: prevalence. *Social Psychiatry* 1: 124–37.

Misiaszek J, Dooling J, Gieseke M et al. (1985) Diagnostic consideration in deaf patients. *Comprehensive Psychiatry* 26(6): 513–21.

Perner J, Frith U, Leslie AM, Leekam S (1989) Exploration of the autistic child's theory of mind: knowledge, belief, and communication. *Child Development* 60(3): 689–700.

Premack D, Woodruff G (1978) Does the chimpanzee have a theory of mind? *Behavioural and Brain Sciences* 4: 515–26.

Reed T, Peterson C (1990) A comparative study of autistic subjects' performance at two levels of visual and cognitive perspective taking. *Journal of Autism and Developmental Disorders* 20(4): 555–68.

Schopler E (1994) A statewide program for the treatment and education of autistic and related communication handicapped children (TEACHH). *Psychoses and Pervasive Developmental Disorders* 3(7): 91–103.

Swaans-Joha BC (1991) *Research Project Mental Health Problems Among Deaf People and Mental Health Care*. Proceedings of the Second International Congress of the European Society for Mental Health and Deafness, Namur, La Bastide, 9–11 May 1991.

Swettenham J, Baron-Cohen S, Gomez JC, Walsh S (1996) What's inside a person's head? Conceiving of the mind as a camera helps children with autism develop an alternative theory of mind. *Cognitive Neuropsychiatry* 1: 73–88.

Tantum D (2000) Psychological disorder in adolescents with Asperger's syndrome. *Autism* 4(1): 47–62.

Volkmar FR, Cohen DJ (1991) Comorbid association of autism and schizophrenia. *American Journal of Psychiatry* 148(12): 1705–7.

Wing L (1997) Asperger's syndrome: management requires diagnosis (editorial). *Journal of Forensic Psychiatry* 8: 253–7.

Wing L, Gould J (1979) Severe impairments of social interaction and associated abnormalities in children: epidemiology and classification. *Journal of Autism and Developmental Disorders* 9(1): 11–29.

Wolff S (1995) *Loners: the Life Path of Unusual Children*, London, Routledge.

World Health Organization (1992) *The ICD-10 Classification of Diseases Clinical Descriptions and Guidelines*, Geneva, World Health Organization.

9

Challenging Behaviours and Deaf Older Adults

DAVID M. FELDMAN AND KRISTYN ECK

INTRODUCTION

The elderly population in America is expected to more than double over the next half century. The culturally Deaf[1] older adult population is also expected to grow at around the same rate. At present, there appears to be a general lack of preparation for the provision of competent and quality services related to the challenges that arise when working with this unique population (Feldman, 2004). This chapter will outline the demographics and socio-economic experiences of the Deaf older adult. It will also attempt to explore some of the more challenging behaviours that may arise for caregivers and mental health professionals when working with both the Deaf older adult and professionals untrained in Deaf-related issues.

DEMOGRAPHICS

Population statistics published by the Gallaudet Research Institute in 1994 suggest that the elderly deaf and hard-of-hearing population

---

[1] 'The use of Deaf for culturally Deaf and deaf for audiologically deaf is now standard in the field of deafness' (Glickman, 2003, p. 17). 'The capitalization of the word "Deaf" is often used to denote an identification of an individual with the Deaf community. This implies a linguistic and cultural understanding, and comfort in being identified as Deaf' (Paul and Jackson, 1993, p. 74).

Deafness and Challenging Behaviour: The 360° Perspective. Edited by S. Austen and D. Jeffery
© 2007 John Wiley & Sons Ltd

totalled more than 11 million and made up about 29.1% of the population of all elderly people in the United States (Holt and Hotto, 1994). Additionally, a 1989 study predicts that the demand for services by deaf and hard-of-hearing older adults will continue to grow, exceeding both the current demand for services and what is currently available (Brown *et al.*, 1989; Hotchkiss, 1989).

HISTORY AND ITS EFFECT ON DEAF OLDER ADULTS

In past decades, the typical attitude of hearing people towards Deaf people has been devaluative and discriminatory, often causing Deaf people to feel inadequate and inferior to hearing peers. Deafness was viewed as a pathologic condition to be corrected by acquiring skills designed to achieve the goal of imitating the majority (i.e. speech/lip-reading, hearing aids) (Gulati, 2003; Lane, 1990). Attitudes that influenced perceptions of deafness in years past would have likely left a lasting impression on Deaf older adults of today. Deaf older adults who experienced this oppression during their developmental and younger adult years often felt themselves to be 'outsiders' in the hearing world, and as members of an 'inferior' group similar to the perceptions of other minorities (Higgins, 1980; Marschark, 1993). Early publications on deafness (Mykelbust, 1950; Peet, 1856) show an adherence to this idea, and reflect how deafness has been long viewed by various professions in this manner. These earlier views would have most affected today's Deaf older adults, their parents and grandparents, and past generations of the hearing general public who were educated on paternalistic portrayals of deafness (Feldman, 2004).

It has been suggested that Deaf people who are born deaf, or have been deaf most of their lives, manifest a certain degree of adjustment and coping ability that develops throughout life in response to stigma, discrimination and social isolation (Becker, 1980; Tidball, 1986). Although this kind of adjustment does not imply an inability to age successfully, it does suggest that cohort effects, as well as the history of the individual and Deaf community, should be examined when discussing client behaviour. Today's Deaf older adult who grew up without the protection of such legislation as the Americans with Disabilities Act 1990, and the required accommodations therein, would have experienced a greater degree of discrimination and oppression than the current younger Deaf adults. Earlier developmental experiences may also shape the perceptions of the hearing professional, who may have grown up with these very paternalistic portrayals and childlike illustrations of deafness and of Deaf people (Feldman, 2004).

Deaf workers, before legislative changes, have generally had less employment opportunities and have earned less than their hearing counterparts (Lane *et al.*, 1996). This situation puts the elderly person at risk for mental health problems for two reasons. First, the Deaf older adult who is economically disadvantaged may not be financially able to afford important goods and services such as recreation, entertainment, transportation or education. These activities are often considered necessary for mental health (e.g. social status, avoidance of isolation and personal growth (Butler *et al.*, 1998)). Second, in countries where mental health services are not provided by the state, the Deaf older adult who has a mental health problem might not be able to afford the costs out of pocket for treatment, which may not be covered, or only partially covered, by medical insurance.

Increased accessibility in the workplace has led to a shift in the economic status for Deaf people and created an economic base greater than has been previously experienced. However, this shift applies mostly to younger Deaf people and, in general, has had less of an effect on the older Deaf population (Feldman, 2004). This group worked primarily in manual labour or low-skill jobs providing low-to-moderate pay and which offered little or no protection against exploitation (Lane *et al.*, 1996).

MENTAL HEALTH SERVICES FOR DEAF OLDER ADULTS

According to Feldman (2004), those providing services to Deaf older adults typically fit into one of three categories:

1. mental health professionals who have training in gerontology but who have little or no experience with Deaf people or ability to communicate directly with Deaf clientele
2. members of the Deaf community itself (or individuals who have standing in the Deaf community) who have experience working with Deaf older adults but lack any academic or formal training in any mental health field
3. mental health professionals who have the training and communication skills in working with Deaf people but who have no training in the area of gerontology.

CASE STUDIES

To illustrate the challenging behaviours that may commonly arise in the evaluation and care of Deaf older adults, the following cases are presented[2] of some of the more common challenging behaviours that have come up during our years in practice. As will be demonstrated through these case studies, the challenging behaviour is often a matter of cultural or linguistic misunderstanding, rather than actual pathology.

Ms A

With the limited number of nursing homes or assisted living facilities specifically for older Deaf adults, the majority of those who need special care often find themselves placed in 'hearing' facilities, and quite often are the only Deaf resident. One of the biggest challenges to Deaf residents in this situation is communication itself. Coupled with that is a lack of understanding on the part of administration and staff related to Deafness (culture, assistive technology, etc.) that can make the behaviours of the Deaf resident appear difficult and challenging.

Ms A was the only Deaf resident in a nursing home. Neither the staff nor other residents could sign or had any experience with Deaf people. Ms A was 73 years old, with some college education and no psychiatric history. She had worked most of her life as a homemaker and had no children. She had always been active in the Deaf community and attended Deaf clubs and a 'Deaf' church. A week after her arrival into the home, staff noticed some behaviour, which was documented as 'acting-out', and she was labelled as 'a difficult resident'. A Mini Mental Status Exam (which has to date not been adapted for use with Deaf older adults) administered by a nurse, with no background in Deafness or signing ability, yielded a score of 9/30 (severely impaired).

Staff had noted that she would steal from the kitchen, isolate herself from other residents and staff, refuse to participate in group activities and 'take things' from other residents. The major complaint related to an incident of 'assaultive behaviour' towards a staff member. The staff had become frustrated with Ms A's behaviours and had already begun

---

[2] As some of the cases presented here are still active, details have been changed or altered in order to protect confidentiality.

to make plans for her to be placed in a more restrictive environment[3]. Before the final plans were laid for her transfer, an attempt was made to consult with a professional with training and experience working with Deaf older adults. On the initial meeting with Ms A, she was interviewed for approximately 45 minutes. Nursing home staff were also interviewed during this visit.

The reports of the staff and Ms A's statements were very similar. Ms A did 'admit' to stealing from the kitchen, taking things from other residents, being isolative, and even to assaulting a staff member. It was noted that (1) the motivation behind her actions was quite different than what was interpreted by staff and (2) these staff interpretations of her behaviours were due to cultural and linguistic misunderstanding, rather than defiance. It became clear that she really did not understand the rules of the house, as no interpreter was provided for the staff's explanations. Ms A was, in fact, 'stealing' from the kitchen because she didn't realise that after a certain time residents were not permitted in that area. The item that she would attempt to take from the other residents was the remote control for the TV, as she wanted to turn on the closed captioning. She admitted to being in her room most of the time because she could not communicate with staff or residents and did not see much point in going into common areas. As for the assault incident, Ms A stated that she had been shaken awake by an unknown woman in the middle of the night and had protected herself. The unknown woman was a staff member who had come to get Ms A for her shower early one morning. Staff had changed the shower schedule and stated they had attempted to communicate this to Ms A. That morning the staff member knocked on her door; when Ms A did not respond, she knocked again, and then she entered her room to find Ms A asleep. The staff member called out her name, and then again louder. When there was no response, she began to tap and shake Ms A. Ms A, who was, by her own admission, 'confused', tried to push her away. A brief struggle ensued.

Certainly, Ms A behaviours were a challenge to the nursing home. However, the root of the problems was the lack of ability to communicate and also basic cultural misunderstanding. The nursing home was in all respects unprepared for a Deaf resident. Unfortunately, very few assisted living facilities or nursing homes have staff that have training in working with Deaf residents or assistive technology specific for Deaf needs.

---

[3] Transfer to a nursing home specific for Deaf residents was not an option.

Much of this situation was resolved by educating the staff. They proved to be very interested in providing a more accommodating environment for Ms A. Interpreters were provided for all 'house meetings'. Captioning was turned on in all common room TVs, a flashing door alarm was set up in her room and a telecommunications device for the Deaf (TDD) was purchased. Special arrangements were made with a local Deaf church for her to attend services and other activities. Once the staff were made more aware of her needs, and she was provided with outside social activities, the nursing home was better able to help Ms A adjust.

Ms B

Cases of cultural misunderstanding and linguistic incompetence are not limited to nursing home staff. Often those in health professions with little or no experience in working with Deaf people find themselves, and their training, to be challenged by the Deaf patient. Lack of training, no language ability and a general misunderstanding of the Deaf patient's culture sets up the clinician for failure and will lead to the patient being misdiagnosed and referred for inappropriate treatment.

Ms B was 79 years old and had been living alone in her own home since her husband died. She attended a residential school for the Deaf, had been active in the Deaf community and, as far as the available records indicated, had never had a mental illness, seen a mental health professional or been prescribed psychotropic medication.

Ms B's family members had noticed some odd behaviour. Ms B had been hiding her laundry in rubbish bags in the basement. She had begun to wear her last set of dirty clothes day after day. Ms B had also cut all the wires in her home that were connected to the doorbell or phone. It was felt by the family that she needed to see a mental health professional for observation. She was brought, with minimal explanation, to a local hospital where she was placed on the psychiatric ward.

During her stay, she was examined by the hospital psychiatrist and a social worker. No interpreter was provided as the social worker had taken a sign language class several years prior and she and the psychiatrist felt that her skill level, along with additional writing back and forth, would be sufficient for communication. After the examination the pair diagnosed Ms B as schizophrenic and recommended she should be placed on antipsychotic medication and transferred to a state psychiatric hospital. Much of this diagnosis was attributed to Ms B's admission that she cut the phone cords because the 'ringing' bothered her. The psychiatrist concluded that this was evidence of auditory hallucination and so, coupled with her other bizarre behaviours, enough to warrant a psychotic disorder diagnosis. Not convinced that this was an appropriate recommendation, her family requested a second opinion.

During the interview with Ms B, she was found to be pleasant and cooperative, somewhat dishevelled and excited that someone was there to see her who could sign. It was quickly realised that several mistakes and misinterpretations had been made on the part of the psychiatrist and social worker. While Ms B reluctantly admitted to hiding her laundry, she explained that she had forgotten how to use her washing machine and was too embarrassed to tell anyone. As for the auditory hallucination, the psychiatrist and social worker, unfamiliar with Deaf culture assumed that the sound of the ringing was bothering her. They did not realise, with their lack of knowledge of Deaf culture, that Ms B was referring to the flashing light alarm system she had set up in her home. She had become annoyed with having the lights flashing, for voice phone calls she could not respond to, and so cut the cords. Although these behaviours are certainly examples of poor judgement and memory impairment, there was little support for a schizophrenic diagnosis. Subsequent psychological testing was suggestive of mild dementia, and Ms B was returned to her home with family supervision.

The lack of familiarity of the hospital staff in the area of Deaf culture and the assumption that a 'sign class' and 'writing back and forth' were efficient means of communication led to an obvious misdiagnosis and treatment recommendations that were inappropriate. Even if the hospital had provided an interpreter, it remains unlikely that the psychiatrist and social worker would have been able to comprehend all the nuances of Deaf culture in order to have been able to ask the right questions, fully understand the answers and in turn make an accurate diagnosis and appropriate treatment plans.

Mr C

Mr C, a 71 year-old Deaf male, was placed in an assisted living facility following a decision made by his son and daughter-in-law. He had no psychiatric or substance abuse history, was a high-school graduate and worked in a skilled trade for most of his adult life. He had always been active in the Deaf community where he attended a residential school for the Deaf, participated in social functions at Deaf clubs and was active in Deaf sports. Mr C had been living with his son and daughter-in-law and their children for the last year following the death of his wife and the sale of his home and car. All of the family members were hearing and his son only had limited signing ability. During this time, Mr C's behaviours became progressively worse. Mr C was described by his son as often moody, defiant and rude, which were not characteristics described to him before the move. Mr C had become increasingly hostile and angry towards his son and daughter in-law, based on what he described as their control over his life and his loss of freedom. They would often argue, which would typically end in Mr C slamming doors and leaving the house for hours at a time. The perspective of the son and daughter-in-law was that Mr C was demanding too much of their time, behaving impulsively and exhibiting angry outbursts.

As he was only able to communicate through his son, Mr C felt frustrated by the lack of communication and socialisation at the home, and his outbursts were directly related to this situation. During most of the day, his son was away at work, leaving Mr C isolated and often confused about the day-to-day activities and events of the household. He stated that on some days he would come out of his room to find the house empty, and as he had no car would sit bored for much of the day. Frustrated, he would confront the daughter-in-law when she returned home, and make demands to be taken someplace. The daughter-in-law could typically not understand his request and often had other responsibilities that did not allow her to chauffer Mr C. As things became worse, he would spend most of his time in his room, stopped bathing, rarely ate and glaring at whatever family members he would happen to come across in the home. It was believed at that time that Mr C was suffering from dementia.

Frustrated and exhausted, the son and daughter-in-law made the difficult decision that his current behaviours required more care than they could provide and the search for an assisted living environment began. The son found that they were living in an area that had an assisted living home with a separate Deaf programme, and arrangements were made for placement. Mr C had a difficult first week and was less than enthusiastic about his new placement. However, after a short time his attitude began to change and it was observed by staff that he was not behaving like the person described by the son and daughter-in-law. Mr C was quite reasonable, was courteous to staff and other residents and demonstrated no angry outbursts or difficulties following rules. He ate regularly and his grooming improved drastically. During regular visits with the family, he appeared to be getting along well, and both the son and daughter-in-law commented on how much he had changed in attitude, behaviour and appearance. Socially, Mr C was active in almost every programme that was offered. He spent most of his time in the common areas and was usually seen with other residents. The idea that he was demented was soon dismissed.

The change in the behaviour of Mr C seems to have been a result of a change in his environment rather than therapeutic intervention. Mr C adapted to the initial change in his living arrangements as well as most residents and very quickly became more active and social. For this previously independent and active Deaf older adult, who was no longer able to participate in social activities while in the family home, the transfer to an assisted living facility with other Deaf older adults and signing staff was a positive experience. Mr C was able to return to the lifestyle he had previously known, with only a few adjustments in living arrangement, and his frustrations and behavioural outbursts were eliminated.

Many Deaf older adults have family members with limited signing ability, and this can create stress on both the Deaf older adult and their family when they come to live in the family home, especially for previously active and social individuals. This is not to suggest that Mr C's family, or any other family in a similar situation, is wrong to allow an older family member to reside in their home. In fact, with so few Deaf facilities there are often few or no other choices, and the family home may be the best option for the Deaf older adult. What is important in these situations is that the Deaf older adult's past lifestyle, cultural preferences and ability for social activity are evaluated. Behaviours that might challenge families without the means to adequately provide for all the needs of their Deaf elders may find themselves faced with a difficult situation and frustration for everyone involved.

CONCLUSION

It seems clear from the several case studies that have been noted here that there are several issues related to the challenging behaviours of the Deaf older adult. However, as demonstrated, what is sometimes described as a challenging behaviour is often more the result of misunderstanding than intentional or dementia-based defiance. These 'behaviours' become especially evident when communication is limited or nonexistent. Professionals who have little or no training of how to work with Deaf people, cannot sign at a sufficient level and become involved in the diagnosis and treatment of the Deaf older adult may misinterpret behaviours or even manifest negative behaviour as a result of cultural incompetence (Feldman, 2005). Certainly, Deaf older adults, as we have seen in these cases, present challenges to professionals, staff and caretakers; however, the challenge is often making sure that qualified personnel are used and Deaf older adults are provided with quality services.

When the environment is supportive of Deaf culture, Deaf older adults whose behaviour has been challenging will likely adjust more successfully. Positive environmental factors may alleviate many of the stressors that can manifest as 'challenging behaviour' issues. For example, it was the availability of professionals with training in working with Deaf older adults and access to other Deaf residents that alleviated the stress in the third case. The home environment was less accommodating, and appropriate placement appears to have been in the assisted living facility. Social activity and communication have an influence on behaviour and the lack of these can result in the manifestation of more negative and challenging behaviours. A home environment, though caring and supportive, may be too limiting especially when the Deaf older adult is faced with few family members that sign and has no access to peer social interaction. Considering the isolation experienced by Deaf older adults who can no longer travel to Deaf community events, placement in a Deaf environment is likely to be preferred.

The education of current and future professionals of the potential challenges that may arise with their Deaf older clientele is fast becoming an extremely important issue in the provision of mental health services for Deaf people. Education and training should focus on the needs of Deaf older adults from both the mental and physical aspects of health. Cultural and technological issues related to service provision are likely to be important related factors. Mental health professionals should also consider that Deaf older adults may be uncomfortable expressing their preferences and have difficulty understanding the technical jargon often used by mental health professionals (Feldman, 2004). Thus, it is up to the professional to familiarise themselves of the needs of Deaf older adults to ensure appropriate and quality mental health services and to be better able to assess the nature of the challenging behaviour.

REFERENCES

Americans with Disabilities Act (1990) 42 USCA http://www.usdoj.gov/crt/ada/adahom1.htm, accessed 23 March 2006.

Becker G (1980) *Growing Old in Silence,* Berkeley, University of California Press.

Brown S, Hotchkiss D, Allen T, Schien J, Adams D (1989) *Current and Future Needs of the Hearing Impaired Elderly Population*, Washington, Gallaudet Research Institute.

Butler R, Lewis M, Sunderland T (1998) *Aging and Mental Health*, Boston, Allyn and Bacon.

Feldman D (2004) Concerns and considerations in mental health practice with culturally deaf older adults. *Journal of the American Deafness and Rehabilitation Association* 37(3): 23–38.

Feldman D (2005) Behaviors of mental health practitioners working with culturally deaf older adults. *Journal of the American Deafness and Rehabilitation Association* 39(2): 31–54.

Glickman N (2003) Cultural affirmative mental health treatment for deaf people: what it looks like and why it is essential. In Glickman N, Gulati S (eds), *Mental Health Care for Deaf People*, Mahwah, NJ, Lawrence Erlbaum, pp. 1–32.

Gulati S (2003) Psychiatric care of culturally deaf people. In Glickman N, Gulati S (eds), *Mental Health Care for Deaf People*, Mahwah, NJ, Lawrence Erlbaum, pp. 33–108.

Higgins P (1980) *Outsiders in A Hearing World*, London, SAGE.

Holt J, Hotto S (1994) *Demographic Aspects of Hearing Impairment: Questions and Answers* (3rd edn.), Washington, Gallaudet University Press.

Hotchkiss D (1989) *The Hearing Impaired Elderly Population: Estimation, Projection and Assessment*, Washington, Gallaudet Research Institute.

Lane H (1990) Cultural and infirmity models of deaf Americans. *Journal of the Academy of Rehabilitative Audiology* 23: 11–26.

Lane H, Hoffmeister R, Bahan B (1996) *A Journey into the Deaf World*, San Diego, DawnSignPress.

Marschark M (1993) *Psychological development of deaf children*, Oxford, Oxford University Press.

Myklebust H (1950) *Your Deaf Child: A Guide for Parents*, Springfield, IL, Charles C. Thomas.

Paul P, Jackson D (1993) *Towards a Psychology of Deafness: Theoretical and Empirical Perspectives*, New York, Allyn and Bacon.

Peet H (1856) On the legal rights and responsibilities of the deaf and dumb. *American Journal of Insanity* 26(2): 97–171.

Reagan T (1990) Cultural considerations in the education of deaf children. In Moores D, Meadows-Orlans K (eds), *Educational and Developmental Aspects of Deafness*, Washington, Gallaudet University Press, pp. 73–80.

Tidball L (1986) A study in the coping strategies developed by older adults who have been deaf since adolescence and possible application of the strategies to the aging process. Doctoral dissertation, University of Nebraska.

PART III
Managing
Challenging Behaviour

10

De-escalation and Deafness: Seeing the Signs?

DAVE JEFFERY AND SALLY AUSTEN

INTRODUCTION

The approximately 70 000 deaf British Sign Language (BSL) users in the UK have at least the same rate of mental health problems as hearing people (Austen, in press). Specifically, according to Meadow (1981) deaf people have a three-times-higher rate of behaviour disorder than hearing people. In this chapter, recommendations are made for maximising effective practice with deaf people who exhibit challenging behaviour. Recent guidance from the National Institute for Clinical Excellence (NICE) has ensured that de-escalation has become fundamental to managing actual or potential aggression (NICE, 2005a). As such, if we are to apply such guidance, considerations must be made as to how de-escalation skills and constructs can be maximised when working with angry deaf service users.

We argue that de-escalation is often unnecessarily sacrificed to the more physical intervention of restraint or to the chemical intervention of PRN (*pro re nata* or 'when necessary') medication. We also describe how methodology and interventions developed for hearing people can be adapted for use with deaf people with behavioural problems.

In addressing reasons why deaf people might be angry, it is reasoned that knowing the service user as an individual and understanding their

Deafness and Challenging Behaviour: The 360° Perspective. Edited by S. Austen and D. Jeffery
© 2007 John Wiley & Sons Ltd

cultural experience are the most important factors in de-escalation. The authors have identified key themes in de-escalation, which highlight possible variants and issues in working with deaf people.

ANGER

Anger is a basic human emotion, which is often associated with aggressive and violent behaviours. Goleman (1996) describes the short-term energising effects of anger as responsible for making it one of the most potent and seductive emotions that we possess. While it does appear to be the mood that we fail to consistently control, Kassinove and Tafrate (2003) believe that aggressive behaviours are not inevitable results of anger. They also note that, while healthcare professionals do not generally share the same emotional experiences as their service users, anger is exceptional. In brief, when our service users get angry, we tend to get angry too.

Zillman (1979) links anger to the individual's sense of endangerment. Fear, threat and anger (the subjective experiences of endangerment) arise within the context of ill thinking (psychosis), limited thinking (learning disability) or well thinking. Anger does not present uniformly. Muir-Cochrane (2003) describes the many guises of anger as:

- intense distress
- pacing
- gritting or grinding teeth
- increased energy
- agitation
- change in tone of voice (raised or lowered)
- raised or lowered eyebrows
- flushed face
- withdrawal
- staring
- fatigue
- clenched fists

CULTURAL MODELS OF ANGER

Anger is not perceived consistently across different cultures (Wierzbicka, 1999). Deaf culture, enshrined in the use of native sign languages, differs in some ways from the equivalent hearing cultures. Thus, English and signed definitions of 'anger' may not be linguistically or emotionally synonymous (Williams and Austen, 2000).

Emotion can be seen as a unique way of understanding culture (Wierzbicka, 1999). It reflects and perpetuates the value and meaning attached to it by the culture in which it is generated. For example, anger is often perceived negatively in Britain and is consciously suppressed through the setting of social standards of behaviour and legislation (Bellah *et al.*, 1985). This may not be the same for other countries or cultures. Anger can alternatively be seen as an emotion that is useful, as instructive and expressive as any other emotion, that has its place and purpose in helping us regulate our behaviour (Holmes and Holmes, 1999).

DE-ESCALATION

'De-escalation' describes a series of verbal and non-verbal behaviours aimed at diffusing anger so that it does not escalate into violence. Anger rather than aggression should be the starting point of de-escalation. Unfortunately, the common association between de-escalation and aggression management means that aggression is seen as the inevitable consequence of anger and intervention is often delayed until challenging behaviour occurs.

In care settings, anger becomes more problematic the longer it remains unidentified, unchecked and unchannelled. Early awareness of anger (the service user's and one's own) allows staff and service users to work collaboratively to diffuse anger where and when individuals have more control and reasoning.

A multitude of variables will determine whether anger results in challenging behaviour. However, the staff member's role in de-escalation is crucial. Anger and aggressive crises can be fuelled or arrested by the verbal and non-verbal behaviour of staff.

CULTURAL MODELS OF DE-ESCALATION

Culture has been recognised as an important variable within de-escalation (Paterson *et al.*, 1998; Bowie, 1996), but definitive guidance or a comprehensive framework as to how this can be realistically applied is lacking. Cultural oppression is a potential catalyst for anger, confrontation and rebellion (Fanon, 1961). More recently, fuelled by the inquiry into the unfortunate death of David 'Rocky' Bennett, where the lack of respect for cultural identity contributed to a catalogue of questionable practices (Blofield *et al.*, 2003), culturally cogent interventions are fast becoming an expectation within the National Health Service (National Institute for Mental Health in England, 2004).

According to Zoucha and Husted (2000), individuality can be sacrificed in the development of culturally congruent care packages. However, the authors would argue that the absence of a culture-specific framework within a contentious area such as aggression management is just as unethical.

PREVENTION OF AGGRESSION IN DEAF PEOPLE

The clinician's role in de-escalation is to find out and change what is making the service user angry. Successful de-escalation can only be achieved by **knowing** the service user: as an individual and as a member of one or more cultural groups. The assumption is that it is usually the angry person who has the 'problem'. Alternatively, by getting to know them as a person and their beliefs about situations, it could become apparent that the cause lies with the staff, the service provision or with society.

CULTURAL KNOWLEDGE OF THE SERVICE USER

For those working in the field of deafness, the concept of disparate hearing and deaf cultures is second nature. The subtle differences between those who identify with the deaf, Deaf or deafened communities are acknowledged (Austen and Coleman, 2004). Whether deafness is viewed by the service user or the staff as either a disability or a cultural lifestyle choice, it is important that de-escalation is planned with respect to both diversity subgroups: disability and culture. The choice to use sign language as the preferred language for anger-management sessions may represent a cultural phenomenon, but the fact that the service user cannot hear a shouted request to calm down demonstrates the need for services to be adapted to the needs of people with disabilities. The oppression and discrimination of people with disabilities and people from minority cultures is common (RNID, 1998).

Cultural Access

Cultural oppression can lead to anger (Fanon, 1961). According to Harris *et al.* (1995), deaf people tend to earn less, have less-skilled jobs and have more difficulties accessing higher education. Deaf people also have poorer access to general health and mental health services (Department of Health, 2005). In summary, in a predominantly hearing world, being deaf results in oppression and discrimination (RNID, 1998).

Services that are staffed by hearing people and that do not specifically provide services for deaf people are often criticised for failing to provide equality of service for deaf service users. However, even services that pride themselves on targeting deaf populations may replicate the oppressive conditions of the general hearing world. While it is not feasible that all healthcare staff learn to sign, it is realistic to expect that all staff that come into contact with deaf service users have 'Deaf awareness', i.e. they appreciate Deaf culture and how to work with a sign language interpreter. However, this is not always the case, even in facilities advertised as being able to treat deaf people with anger problems.

The less deaf aware (an awareness of Deaf culture and/or an understanding of sign language) staff are, the more likely it is that they may misinterpret a deaf person's innocuous behaviour as challenging behaviour. For example, within Deaf culture a certain degree of directness, more than in hearing culture, can be used without giving offence. For example, 'I don't like your glasses. They make you look like an owl' would be considered rude in hearing culture and not so in Deaf culture. Furthermore, within Deaf culture a greater degree of touch and body contact can be used before it implies assault or personal intrusion.

Communication Breakdown

Communication is crucial to assessing and knowing a person. In the absence of easy communication with a service user, it is sometimes possible to take a history from family or previous professionals, but this is far from ideal. Communicating directly with the deaf service user may not be easy. There are extremely few deaf professionals, whether in the health, probation, education or mental health fields, and it is rare that hearing professionals can sign. Likewise, few hearing parents of deaf children sign.

In the absence of people who have signing skills, deaf people have to communicate in their second language (speech and lip-reading) and may find this frustrating. Deaf people's general skills in lip-reading will depend on many factors such as degree and onset of deafness and educational experience. During specific conversations, lip-reading efficacy will depend on factors dependent on the deaf person, such as degree of fatigue, interest in and previous knowledge of the subject as well as factors dependent on the hearing person: the speed and rhythm of their voice, their use of facial expression, the presence of facial hair, such as a beard, and distracting features such as sparkly earrings. The environment will also affect lip-reading: appropriate lighting, the absence of visual distractions such a busy wallpaper, activity within eyeshot or distance between the two people communicating. Lip-reading efficacy is also dependent on the emotional state of the deaf person. In situations of heightened arousal, for example when angry or frightened, lip-reading would be particularly difficult. Even good lip-readers will miss parts of what is said directly to them. The greatest potential for miscommunication, however, is that lip-reading is only possible face to face. This means that in the average day much of the surrounding conversations, TV broadcasts, salutations, instructions and throw-away comments are missed.

Even when the professional and the service user are communicating in the same language, there is still the potential for communication breakdown, particularly if the deaf person has minimal language skills and/or poor educational experience. An unproven myth that signing to deaf children inhibits speech has resulted in many hearing parents being advised not to sign to their deaf children, which for some children results in language deprivation. This in turn has long-term repercussions for the development of Theory of Mind, reasoning skills and learning, all of which are crucial to the understanding of others' behaviours, one's own behaviour and society's boundaries.

Role-Modelling and Poor Boundary Setting

As children grow up, boundary setting is crucial to future appropriate behaviour. Where the person giving the instructions has little sign language, instructions are often given in a concrete, oversimplified and directive manner, rather than the abstract or complex explanations that would have been used with an equivalent hearing child (Schlesinger and Meadow, 1972). While some of our learning is through direct tuition, most of what we acquire is learnt incidentally.

That which we 'overhear' provides crucial information about both fact and process. For deaf children who do not hear verbal, or see signed, explanation, reasoned debate is impossible to observe and therefore learn. In this situation, visual role models gain a greater influence such that those TV characters or local heroes that stand out become the guides to the child's behaviour. We have seen in the example provided by the second service user in the opening chapter of this book that the 'hearing gang' with all its violence and glamour was extremely attractive over the 'boring' lifestyle that mixing with deaf people and behaving well provided.

Alongside parents and teachers, the criminal justice system is also responsible for boundary setting. It seems that the burdensome procedures involved in prosecuting deaf people guilty of crimes, e.g. arranging appropriately skilled interpreters, and a rather paternalistic pity for them has resulted in a degree of overprotection and a lack of prosecutions (Hindley *et al.*, 2000). Such poor boundary setting and the lack of consistent consequences will result in increasingly challenging behaviour.

INDIVIDUAL KNOWLEDGE OF THE SERVICE USER

Despite sharing common experiences such as discrimination, isolation and misunderstanding, deaf people should also be recognised as individuals with unique experiences that may or may not be related to their deafness.

Anger is often pathologised or assumed to be associated with mental illness. However, there is an extremely limited pool of professionals capable of adequately assessing deaf people with additional needs and they often become part of a system (school, prison or hospital) without ever being fully assessed. Assessment of cognitive functioning (intelligence, memory, attention, Theory of Mind etc.), mental state and language (with particular reference to comprehension) is crucial. Resources are often such that the actual assessment falls short of the ideal assessment, but this should not detract us from aiming high. When Meadow (1981) found that behaviour disorder was three times as common in deaf than hearing people, she was referring to community samples, which means that the rate of behaviour disorder is likely to be even higher in psychiatric samples.

For some deaf people, their cause of deafness has been associated with an assault on the brain such as meningitis or rubella. Subtle cognitive deficits may be present, which increase the risk of irritability and decrease the ability to inhibit behaviour. Owing to limited psychiatric or neurological services for deaf people and the lack of valid psychometric tests for deaf people, few deaf people have been assessed for such difficulties.

Negative Thinking

It is highly possible for a person to feel victimised in the absence of abuse. Thus, an assessment of not just language but also of the service user's cognitions and beliefs is important. The cognitive behavioural model (Beck *et al.*, 1979) allows investigation of how aggression may have been the result of the subject misinterpreting a particular situation. For example, if staff are not signing, a deaf person may wrongly assume they are talking about him or her. Cognitive frameworks (or schema), negative and positive, are built up as a result of life experience. Whether deaf or hearing, a sense of criticism or the experience of oppression may be associated with an inaccurate interpretation of innocuous comments. For example, the comment 'You have forgotten your glasses' may be perceived as 'You have made a mistake and are stupid'.

NATIONAL GUIDANCE AND DE-ESCALATION

NICE has made clear that de-escalation skills **must** be used before care staff decide to employ physical restraint or use PRN medication (NICE, 2005a). Figure 10.1 illustrates just how intrinsic de-escalation has become in managing a potentially aggressive individual. Relatively little rigorous study has been done in the field of de-escalation, and only recently has there been recognition of the care needs of deaf service users at a point of crisis (Medical Directors Council, 2002; NICE, 2005b). Yet there are only limited levels of study concerning the effectiveness of hearing-based de-escalation strategies and their use with deaf service users (Jeffery and Austen, 2005).

In terms of the NICE overview algorithm de-escalation can be considered an ongoing process. The earlier this process is used, the more effective its potential effect. This is important when we consider the alternative strategies that may be employed once aggression begins to move to a point of crisis. The use of medication to manage anger and aggression is not without its problems and should only be used after de-escalation has proved ineffective. The impact for service users who

Overview algorithm for the short-term management of disturbed/violent behaviour

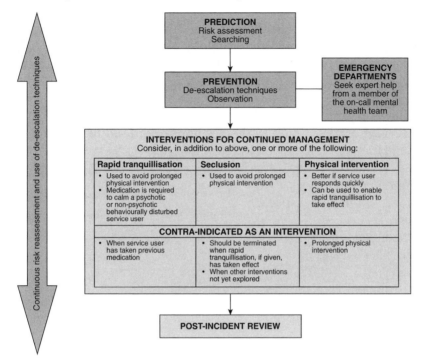

Figure 10.1 The Nice Algorithm, © National Institute for Clinical Excellence (NICE) (2005) *The Short-term Management of Disturbed/Violent Behaviour in In-patient Psychiatric Settings and Emergency Departments.* London: NICE. Available from www.nice.org.uk. Reproduced with permission of National Institute for Health and Clinical Excellence.

receive pharmaceutical intervention in the form of PRN medication or rapid tranquillisation during restraint has potential to outlast the crisis event itself. Unwanted side effects (i.e. sedation), lack of impulse control from the administration of benzodiazepines (Paton, 2002) and a service user's possible future reliance on medication to control their behaviour are strong factors to support de-escalation as the primary intervention. Repeated use of PRN medication can lead the service user to believe that containing his or her behaviour is the responsibility of the staff. If the service user relies on staff for such fundamental control, they are unlikely to learn to regulate their behaviour themselves.

KEY THEMES OF DE-ESCALATION

De-escalation models, with differing theoretic foundations, but informed by an array of psychological, ethological and sociological paradigms, appear to share certain key themes. The authors (Jeffery and Austen, 2005) have applied the key themes that come out of the existing de-escalation programmes, which are specifically designed for working with hearing service users, to working with potentially angry deaf service users. These key themes have been used to generate recommendations to maximise effective practice.

- communication
- stance and personal space
- touch
- eye contact
- face
- voice
- environment

COMMUNICATION

Communication is multifaceted and is integral to most therapeutic approaches to aggression (Thackery, 1987). Communication between hearing people comprises both verbal and non-verbal behaviour, whereas signed and 'non-verbal behaviour' is virtually indistinguishable in communication between people using sign language. Effective sign language involves actions such as movements and expressions of face and body, as well as eye contact (Smith, 1992). Therefore, some behaviours are replicated in both the communication and the therapeutic intervention.

Staff members should endeavour to know the style, preferences and nuances within their service user's language. Particular language styles of individuals may bring specific communication issues. It may be that the deaf person has additional disabilities or limitations that include idiosyncratic or limited language skills. Communication between staff and service user is crucial to de-escalation, as the language style or choice of specific words may be the variable that affects the service user's ability to self-control or otherwise. The authors recommend that a native Deaf signer analyse the intricacies of the emotional content of particular words or signs for each service user on first referral or admission and their favoured words and terms in regards to aggression be noted. The same Deaf staff member could also interview the service user and their family to find out how they perceived previous methods of aggression management, de-escalation or restraint. During an aggressive outburst, both hearing and deaf service users benefit from simple sentences with clear contexts to avoid overloading the angry person with information. This is particularly important with deaf services users who have additional language limitations or difficulties.

Working with Interpreters

Deaf services usually employ both deaf and hearing staff who ideally can sign fluently. However, it is not always the case, and sign language interpreters are sometimes needed in situations of de-escalation. To maximise the effectiveness of the de-escalation, the interpreter should know the service user well, including their particular style of language use. For some service users, the use of the interpreter may highlight their isolated and subservient position and therefore exacerbate the aggression. Alternatively, it may reduce some of the emotional content and the immediacy of the communication between service user and staff and therefore reduce aggressive potential. However, this assumes that the interpreter remains completely impartial throughout the interpreting task, which is unlikely. The interpreter, despite professional codes of conduct, may intentionally or unintentionally alter the translation of angry material in the hope that resolution can be achieved without aggression. They would not be human if they did not. Ways to reduce the interpreter influence needs to be discussed openly in the course of the post-incident debrief. This is discussed further in this book in the chapters pertaining to Deaf staff and interpreters (Chapter 13) and the potential traumatic effect of staff of working with challenging behaviour (Chapter 3).

STANCE AND PERSONAL SPACE

Bowie (1996) reports that when individuals become highly aroused their ability to take in verbal cues is inhibited, which makes them more susceptible to non-verbal methods of communication. This may be magnified in deaf people, whose primary source of information is visual. BSL makes use of stance and posture to relay a person's mood and intention. For example, standing with arms crossed or on hips can be perceived as authoritative or confrontational. Staff must therefore demonstrate neutral stances to avoid misinterpretation.

Stance is more than a representation of feelings or intent, however. It is integral to maintaining safety. While signing, the natural position of the hands is slightly raised. Should a service user become aggressive, the hands can quickly be moved from a signing position to a defensive position. It is usual when signing to stand face to face. However, the authors recommend that staff stand with their body angled at a 45-degree side-on position to the service user, with signing at chest height. This will protect their vulnerable areas from possible assault.

Hildreth *et al.* (1971) suggest that angry people have an increased need for personal space, which can be up to six times the normal level of distance the individual can usually tolerate when calm. For sign language users, lip-readers and deaf/blind people this recommendation may be unworkable. Optimum distance for communication will need to be balanced with the requirements of staff safety.

TOUCH

In order to use touch during de-escalation, one would require an intimate knowledge of each individual service user. Touch in such contexts is often seen as inappropriate and contentious. Patterson *et al.* (1998) believe that touch should be avoided as its outcome is too unpredictable.

Touch is more culturally acceptable within the Deaf world. For example, it is normal to gain the attention of a deaf person by lightly placing a hand on a shoulder or forearm; and touch is crucial to communicate using the Deaf/blind manual alphabet (DBMA). However, touch still needs to be used sensitively, recognising the individual's diversity. In all circumstances, efforts should be taken to get well within the deaf person's visual field before attempting to touch or to communicate. In circumstances where a service user may view staff as protagonists, or be paranoid, anxious or defensive, approach from outside of the visual field is particularly unwise.

EYE CONTACT

In communicating with an angry person, a balance must be achieved between socially appropriate eye contact and staring with perceived provocative intent (Bowie, 1996). Poor eye contact may be seen as dismissive and disrespectful or give signals that imply submission and which could trigger an assault.

Both the delivery and receipt of BSL requires good eye contact. In working with deaf people, using either speech or sign, eye contact will be prolonged. Lane *et al.* (1996) suggest that, within the Deaf community, breaking eye contact during interaction is discourteous. If a sign language interpreter is used, the principal eye contact will be between the service user and interpreter. The hearing person should continue to look at the deaf person throughout the signed and voiced-over responses. This respectfully acknowledges the deaf person as the source of the message and allows the hearing person to observe the deaf service user's types and degree of non-verbal communication.

Occasionally, a service user will choose to respond to the interpreter and not acknowledge the practitioner. This may indicate hostility on the part of the service user. Even though the service user may require the emotional distance from the clinician, it is not appropriate to leave the interpreter with the clinical responsibility of direct communication with the patient. To counteract this, and maximise eye contact between the clinician and service user, the interpreter can position themselves slightly behind or to the side of the clinician. Further discussion about the service user's desire or need to prevent communication with the clinician should be discussed or dealt with by the clinician at a time that they feel is appropriate.

FACE

Basic emotional expression has found commonality in the human face (Ekman and Rosenberg, 1997), and BSL utilises the face to underpin grammatical syntax and reinforce verbs (Lane *et al.*, 1996). The face, expressing the message conveyed in BSL, cannot therefore be taken as indicative of intention without a full understanding of the message that is being conveyed. For example, to describe in sign language the anger and violence of Person A, requires the innocuous signer (Person B) to use their face to portray the angry face and their arms to describe how the angry Person A hit out. The nature of sign language is such that it gets bigger, stronger and more expressive with the greater amount of emotion. Therefore, a deaf Person B, describing an angry Person A, could be mistaken for being angry themselves. Likewise, a staff member without knowledge of its full context coming upon a conversation about someone else's outburst and threats to kill may be inclined to intervene physically. This confirms the importance of maximising communication (between staff as well as between staff and service users) and of having as good a knowledge as possible of the service user.

VOICE

'Voice', in the context of working with deaf people, needs some explanation. Given that many deaf people will neither hear the voice of a staff member nor use their own voice, in BSL the 'voice' refers to the style and content of an interaction. Similarly to spoken English, BSL can communicate containment or panic, calm or hostility. De-escalation should ideally enable staff to 'talk down' an angry deaf service user without risking 'talking down' to them. Clinicians and interpreters must therefore be aware of their 'tone' and be open to instruction and feedback on their communication style from more able signers.

Shouting at a deaf person is ineffective and condescending and the resulting exaggerated mouth shapes limit lip-reading.

ENVIRONMENT

The importance of the environment in the prevention or management of violence is heightened in working with deaf people. Signing requires the physical space for arms and body to move. For staff to physically intervene and to accommodate two emotionally fuelled people signing, corridors need to be wider and rooms bigger. During an argument in signed language, it is almost certain that arms will be moving rapidly. It is therefore important that breakable objects and unhardened glass windows are kept out of reach as much as possible. Breakages are expensive, bad for staff morale and increase a service user's distress.

To allow signing in all areas at all times, lighting should be bright but without being so harsh that it causes eye strain. Visual features are particularly prominent for deaf people; so colours and patterns should be easy on the eyes and window dressings designed to control light input while minimising the flicker of incoming sunlight.

CONCLUSION

Aggression management is a topic full of controversy with the need for ethical practice and cultural cogency high on the agenda. All service users with aggressive behaviours should be managed within frameworks that recognise their specialist and diverse needs. NICE is clear that de-escalation must be attempted before either restraint or PRN medication are considered. It is clear that without the recognition and acknowledgement of cultural identity a 'one size fits all' approach to de-escalation may fail the deaf person at the point of crisis. Such a failure may well result in physical intervention. Given this premise, mental health practitioners have a duty to explore ways to maximise the effectiveness of current approaches, while developing culturally cogent strategies.

This chapter has explored the applicability to deaf people of de-escalation methodology evolved from work with hearing people. Without an awareness of sign language and Deaf culture, the effectiveness of such strategies are compromised. Key themes of various de-escalation frameworks have been highlighted and then adapted in order to maximise their effectiveness when managing aggressive deaf service users. Potential areas of dilemma and suggestions for improving intervention effectiveness have been discussed.

REFERENCES

Austen S (in press) A snapshot of mental health and deafness, *Deaf Worlds*.

Austen S, Coleman E (2004) Controversy in deafness: *Animal Farm* meets *Brave New World*. In Austen S, Crocker S (eds), *Deafness in Mind: Working Psychologically with Deaf People*, London, Whurr, pp. 3–20.

Beck AT, Rush AJ, Shaw BF, Emery G (1979) *Cognitive Therapy of Depression*, Chichester, Wiley.

Bellah RN, Sullivan WM, Tipton SM, Swidler A, Madson RP (1985) *Habits of the Heart: Individualism and Commitment in American Life*, Berkley, University of California Press.

Blofield J, Sallah D, Sashidaran S, Stone R, Struthers J (2003) *Independent Inquiry into the Death of David Bennett HSG (94) 27*, Cambridge, Norfolk, Suffolk and Cambridgeshire Strategic Health Authority Publication.

Bowie V (1996) *Coping With Violence: A Guide for the Human Services* (2nd edn.), London, Whiting.

Department of Health (2005) *Mental Health and Deafness: Towards Equity and Access*, London, TSO.

Ekman P, Rosenberg E (1997) *What the Face Reveals*, New York, Oxford University Press.

Fanon F (1961) *The Wretched of the Earth*, London, Penguin Classics.

Goleman D (1996) *Emotional Intelligence: Why It Can Matter More Than IQ*, London, Bloomsbury.

Harris JP, Anderson JP, Novak R (1995) An outcomes study of cochlear implants in deaf patients: audiologic, economic, and quality-of-life changes. *Archives of Otolaryngology, Head and Neck Surgery* 121(4): 398–404.

Hildreth AM, Derogatis LR, McCusker K (1971) Body buffer zone and violence: a reassessment and confirmation. *The American Journal of Psychiatry* 127(12): 1641–5.

Hindley P, Kitson N, Leach V (2000) Forensic psychiatry and deafness. In Hindley P, Kitson N (eds), *Mental Health and Deafness*, London, Whurr pp. 206–31.

Holmes R, Holmes J (1999) *The Good Mood Guide: How to Embrace Your Pain and Face Your Fears*, London, Orion Mass Market Paperback.

Jeffery D, Austen S (2005) Adapting de-escalation techniques with deaf service users. *Nursing Standard* 19(49): 41–47.

Kassinove H, Tafrate RC (2003) *Anger Management: The Complete Treatment Guidebook for Practitioners* (3rd edn.), Atascadero, CA, Impact.

Lane H, Hoffmeister R, Bahan B (1996) *A Journey into the Deaf-World*, San Diego, Dawn Sign Press.

Meadow KP (1981) Studies of behaviour problems of deaf children. In Stein L, Mindel E, Jabaley T (eds), *Deafness and Mental Health*, New York, Grune and Stratton, pp. 3–22.

Medical Directors Council (2002) *Reducing the Use of Seclusion and Restraint: Lessons from the Deaf and Hard of Hearing Communities: A Technical Report.* Alexandra, VA: National Association of State Mental Health Program Directors.

Muir-Cochrane E (2003) The person who is aggressive or violent. In Barker P (ed), *Psychiatric and Mental Health Nursing: The Craft of Caring*, London, Arnold, pp. 274–80.

National Institute for Clinical Excellence (2005a) *The Short-term Management of Disturbed/Violent Behaviour in In-patient Psychiatric Settings and Emergency Departments: Guideline 25*, London, NICE.

National Institute for Clinical Excellence (2005b) *The Short-term Management of Disturbed/Violent Behaviour in In-patient Psychiatric Settings and Emergency Departments: Full Report*, London, NICE.

National Institute for Mental Health in England (2004) *Developing Positive Practice to Support the Safe and Therapeutic Management of Aggression and Violence in Mental Health In-patient Settings: Mental Health Policy Implementation Guide*, London, Department of Health.

Paterson B, Leadbetter D, McComish A (1998) De-escalation in the management of aggression and violence. *Nursing Times* 93(36): 58–61.

Paton C (2002) Benzodiazepines and disinhibition: a review. *Psychiatric Bulletin* 26: 460–2.

Royal National Institute for Deaf People (1998) *Breaking the Sound Barrier*, London, Royal National Institute for Deaf People.

Schlesinger HP, Meadow KP (1972) Development or maturity in deaf children. *Exceptional Children* (February): 461–7.

Smith C (1992) *Signs Make Sense: A Guide to British Sign Language*, London, Souvenir Press (Educational and Academic).

Tavris C (1989) *Anger: The Misunderstood Emotion Touchstone*, New York, Simon & Schuster.

Thackery M (1987) *Therapeutics for Aggression: Psychological/Physical Crisis*, New York, Intervention Human Science Press.

Wierzbicka A (1999) *Emotions Across Language and Cultures: Diversity and Universals*, New York, Cambridge University Press.

Williams C, Austen S (2000) Deafness and intellectual impairment: double jeopardy? In Hindley P, Kitson N (eds), *Mental Health and Deafness*, London, Whurr, pp. 99–126.

Zillman D (1979) *Hostility and Aggression*, Hillsdale, NJ, Lawrence Erlbaum.

Zoucha R, Husted GL (2000) The ethical dimensions of delivering culturally congruent nursing and health care. *Issues in Mental Health Nursing* 21(3): 325–40.

11

Showing Restraint: Therapeutic Holding with Deaf People in Crisis

DAVE JEFFERY

In its most elementary sense, to be at liberty – or to be free – means to be unfettered. (Szasz, 1989, p. 6)

INTRODUCTION

There is a recognised need for aggressive service users with mental health problems to be managed within frameworks that recognise their specialist and diverse needs (NICE, 2005). Specific guidance, however, is lacking. Consequently, there is a duty amongst mental health practitioners to rigorously examine generic approaches and gauge their suitability in the care and treatment of those individuals with special needs.

This chapter examines this notion from the viewpoint of caring for deaf service users in mental health crisis and explores intrinsic factors that may negate the use of some physical restraint philosophies and techniques. The author will examine the history and application of restraint in the UK and identify key issues that could impact upon the delivery of culturally cogent practice.

The author considers the term **restraint** value-laden. Therefore the idiom **therapeutic holding** will be applied when discussing culturally

Deafness and Challenging Behaviour: The 360° Perspective. Edited by S. Austen and D. Jeffery
© 2007 John Wiley & Sons Ltd

cogent physical interventions with deaf service users. However, no form of physical intervention can be considered therapeutic in isolation and without recognition of the ethical, legal and professional constructs that determine and govern its use.

ORIGINS OF PHYSICAL RESTRAINT IN THE UK

There is an unfortunate association between restraint and psychiatry. This can be illustrated by Pinel's gesture of unchaining a mentally ill prisoner from the walls of Bicêtre prison and asylum for the insane in eighteenth-century Paris. Once considered recognition of the medicalisation of madness, this act heralded the birth of social conscience in the care of the mentally ill (Szasz, 2003).

Restraint in the UK arose from a different setting. 'Control and Restraint' (C&R) was devised by members of the physical instruction team of the Metropolitan Police as a specialised form of physical intervention to support police officers and the prison service staff. The use of C&R in mainstream psychiatry began with the recommendations of the *Ritchie Inquiry* (Ritchie, 1985). The lack of a recognised aggression management system was considered contributory to the death of Michael Martin in Broadmoor special hospital in 1984. C&R was adapted for use in special hospitals in the absence of other robust methods of managing aggressive behaviour and over a period of ten years found its way into generic mental healthcare facilities throughout the UK. C&R has since become synonymous with restraint per se, yet it is important to note that in this context it is a generic term incorporating systems that do not use pain compliance.

TRAGEDY AND THE AGGRESSION MANAGEMENT RENAISSANCE

The death of Michael Martin may have generated debate and informed a national response, yet it did not prevent further tragedy. In the past fifteen years, several high-profile inquiries into restraint-related deaths in mental health facilities in the UK have questioned both its application and how it is taught (UKCC, 2000). This is not a shame that the UK shares alone. The Citizens Commission on Human Rights (CCHR, 2004) has established that up to 150 restraint-associated deaths occur per annum in the USA. The youngest reported casualty was six years old.

A primary catalyst for the recent aggression management renaissance was the inquiry into the death of David Bennett, who died at the Norvic Clinic, Norwich in 1998 (Blofield *et al.*, 2003). Recommendations from the inquiry arrived following a six-year investigation and collation of data, generating renewed urgency to review the delivery of physical interventions in the UK.

In the hiatus between publication of definitive national guidance (NICE, 2005), the National Institute for Mental Health in England (NIMHE) presented a policy framework aimed at bridging policy-implementation deficits in the management of aggression and violence in mental healthcare settings in the UK (NIMHE, 2004).

Ever on the agenda, polemic and contentious, physical interventions are a sour side of practice. However, it has been agreed that focusing upon the physical skills themselves, without context or underpinning evidence based knowledge, is a recipe for tragedy and abusive practice (Beech, 2001; Gournay, 2001). In this instance, context is established within three distinct areas.

1. ethical context and deafness
2. legal context and deafness
3. professional context and deafness

Each of these areas will be examined in detail, taking into account the implications for managing actual and potential aggression and their subsequent influence upon the practice of caring for the deaf person in crisis.

ETHICAL CONTEXT AND DEAFNESS

Watson puts succinctly the underpinning philosophy that all aggression management approaches must adopt:

> It should be obvious that restricting someone's movement against their wishes is entirely wrong in almost all circumstances (Watson, 2002, p. 31)

The association of madness and human immorality prompted the Quakers to develop mechanical restraint as a method to manage events deemed to be without reason and, as such, an affront to the individual's humanity (Colaizzi, 2005). In essence, no different from the shackles of the Bicêtre, the use of the straitjacket constituted a fundamental shift in the ethical philosophy underpinning the use of restraint: that of an intervention on behalf of the individual's social and moral salvation and for the betterment (or rather protection) of others. This is a concept that has remained in mental health facilities around the world to this day.

There is a danger in accepting without question that which is done to another in the name of the greater good. Much governs the decision to physically hold another person, and in practice this is never clear. Ethical cogence is measured by consideration and application of philosophies that acknowledge and underpin all aspects of the dynamics of the crisis event. This element has been considered missing from traditional approaches to managing aggression (Gournay, 2001).

Tarbuck (1992a) examined the ethical contexts of restraint. In this context, ethics have been defined as:

> indicators and principles within professional groups of what is accepted as correct behaviour when dealing with client groups. (Tarbuck, 1992b, p. 27)

This definition is somewhat misleading. The 'indicators and principles' here relate to C&R, a system devised and set by a group of professionals outside the mental healthcare arena, and without an ethical framework informing its original design. On this basis, the issue of paternalism becomes almost an aside to the main focus of 'controlling' the service user's behaviour.

The concept of paternalism emerged after the publications of deontologist Immanuel Kant and utilitarian John Mill (Beauchamp and Childress, 2001). Deontology, the theory that some actions are obligatory regardless of consequences, and utilitarianism, the notion that the greater good guides any action that is taken, pervade most ethical literature on restraint practice (Hopton, 1995), usually as most ethical scrutiny seeks to justify its use. However, while diametrically opposed, both deontology and utilitarianism advocate that a fundamental facet to ethical doctrine is the promotion of autonomy.

Beauchamp and Childress (2001) developed a series of principles to aid care staff in ethical decision-making. The framework consists of four components: autonomy, beneficence, non-maleficence and justice. It would be useful to consider the ethical issues of therapeutic holding and the deaf person exhibiting challenging behaviour within this existing framework.

Autonomy

Autonomy is concerned with the facilitation of a person's self-governance or independence. The promotion of autonomy is compromised by interventions designed to limit the behaviours or liberties of individuals demonstrating challenging behaviour. The restrictive nature of a restraint process automatically introduces the concept of power once it is applied, and the imbalance of this dynamic can not only perpetuate the crisis event but potentially damage the therapeutic alliance post incident (Sequeira and Halstead, 2002).

Hearing care staff who hold down a deaf person need to be aware of the concept of autonomy, especially when the historical experiences of the Deaf community are considered within the context of cultural oppression and social exclusion. Long-term exposure to basic infringements of self-governance has been affiliated to societal expectations of deafness as a disability, warranting the search for a cure over the promotion of cultural cogence via the exposition of sign language. This has led to the suppression of sign language throughout the ages. An example is illustrated by certain educational establishments who have traditionally punished deaf students for using sign language in class.

It is important that the use of physical interventions acknowledge the need to empower the individual at the earliest opportunity. The obvious way in which to do this is to employ physical skills that promote the use of effective communication in order to facilitate resolution. This would require policies and the endorsement of therapeutic holding skills that do not require a person's wrist to be immobilised using flexion, thus allowing the deaf service user to engage in signed dialogue.

There is some debate concerning the relationship between the use of pain compliance and the influence this may have in the promotion of autonomy. This follows the misguided belief that the service user is in control of the painful stimulus because, it is argued, any pain that is incurred is the result of resisting the wrist locks applied by care staff. Such a skewed rationale is fraught with issues, especially when the notion of autonomous action must be related to the ability of individuals to demonstrate:

> intention, understanding and independence from controlling influences (Paterson, 2005, p. 21)

Beneficence

The notion that every act upon which we embark should be for the common good embodies the beneficence idiom. However, in terms of the application of restraint, what is considered 'common good' is a subjective judgement. Care staff may feel managing challenging behaviours warrants intervention, whereas service users may consider such behaviours as freedom of expression. The traditional C&R perspective, unavoidable to some degree given their origins within facilities designed to contain, rests upon 'controlling' the behaviour and therefore controlling the individual.

Non-maleficence

There is consensus in that any intervention employed should not place its recipient at risk. Non-maleficence, or 'to do no harm', is arguably the most obvious ethical principle when managing challenging behaviour with physical intervention. What is not so clear is the context in which harm occurs. As noted, deaths from unorthodox restraint are not a rarity on a global scale, and these are clear examples of a failure to apply this principle in practice.

The psychological cost to the service user is an area of limited study (Smith, 1995). Those studies that have explored these factors have noted that service users find the restraint experience psychologically challenging, evoking memories of previous experiences, especially for those who have been exposed to sexual abuse (Smith, 1995; Bonner *et al.*, 2002). An emergent theme of research conducted by Bonner *et al.* (2002) suggests that physical interventions that involve pain compliance and perceived negative staff attitudes create a sense of anger and frustration in some service users that in turn promote further problematic behaviours. It is therefore important to consider the impact of physical intervention based upon the person under restraint, not the behaviours that they present.

Justice

Justice must suit the individual and society. Beauchamp and Childress suggest that the ethical tenet encompassed in justice can be interpreted as:

> fair, equitable, and appropriate treatment in light of what is due or owed to persons. (Beauchamp and Childress, 2001, p. 226)

It is argued that the true nature of justice requires a balance between societal benefit and burden and the equitable distribution of such facets to its citizens.

The management of a deaf person in crisis rests upon societal values of an individual's ability or inability to make decisions or choices. The deaf person has often been considered by society as having lower intellect or a disability. While not immediately obvious, prejudicial viewpoints of society at large are a good starting point for service providers to develop appropriate care systems since inequity and lack of cultural cogence are often fuelled by such misconceptions. There is an assumption that being deaf constitutes not having the capacity to control or understand one's own behaviours. As such, interventions have been used that have been designed for hearing service users with challenging behaviours, but justified using this assumption. True equity in practice requires an exploration of elements that are intrinsic to an awareness of Deaf culture and the development of culture-specific systems within both deaf and generic services (Jeffery and Austen, 2005).

When restraining deaf service users, practitioners have often faced a basic dilemma that brings them into direct conflict with ethical doctrines. The act of restricting the use of a Deaf person's hands could be conceived as an act of suppression since sign language becomes a natural casualty of simple mechanics.

As mentioned in Chapter 10, the use of touch is an integral part of Deaf culture. It is used to announce, initiate and establish interaction (Kitson *et al.*, 2000). In limiting the movement of a deaf person's hands, communication becomes reliant upon the powerful messages we send through touch. If the holds that are applied were causing pain or discomfort, it would be of little surprise if the deaf person interprets the restrainer as uncaring and oppressive. The issue here is that the person will not be able to verbally indicate their concerns and is therefore left with limited options to communicate them. It is of little surprise if the person employs further physical activity as a method of dialogue, which the staff could interpret as an escalation of challenging behaviour.

The debate concerning the application of restraint skills that by their nature inflict pain is ongoing. A distinction has been drawn as to its limited value in helping to de-escalate a person's crisis and its ethical validity questioned given the emergence and recognition nationally of holding skills that do not rely on painful stimuli (NICE, 2005).

LEGAL CONTEXT AND DEAFNESS

The act of one person making physical contact with another without invitation or consent places the practitioner within legal parameters. Legal constructs have a primary focus on the action or omissions of individual members of staff during the crisis event. The underpinning philosophy is that of how **reasonable** the decisions to act or not to act were given the service user's behaviour or the situation in which such behaviour occurred. What adds to the confusion is a lack of a legal definition of the term 'reasonable'.

Decisions to intervene are often informed by the **duty of care** practitioners have to the deaf person, other members of staff and other service users in the vicinity. Duty of care exists to underpin the concept of responsibility to another for whom we have a societal obligation. As professional carers, a legal duty of care exists in terms of ensuring that acts (things we do) or omissions (things we don't do) do not expose the service user to harm. This principle is measured against the probable, or reasonably foreseeable, outcome of these factors.

The dilemma here is that restraint is used to manage behaviours which have a probable outcome that may cause harm to others, yet may still cause injury or psychological distress to the person displaying the behaviours. In this instance, the use of restraint would need to be shown to be proportionate to the behaviours being displayed by the service user. This idiom is known as **reasonable force**. The paradox is that if carers consider all aspects challenging behaviour requiring them to immediately intervene lest they be criticised for not doing so this may lead to reactive practice. What is subsequently lost is an individualistic approach to such behaviours and infringements upon a service user's autonomy. It is important that such factors are not sacrificed in the name of defensive practice, especially in view of recent international legislation. Article 3 of the Human Rights Act (HMSO, 1998) has a fundamental impact upon the use of restraint within the context of any act perpetuated towards another individual in the name of care stating it should not involve:

inhumane or degrading treatment or punishment (HMSO, 1998, p. 27)

The loss of liberty imposed by the use of restraint defines the dilemma for service users and care staff alike. In the UK, supportive guidance through the Mental Health Act 1983 assists staff in the process of using minimum restraint to 'intervene' to prevent a crime from occurring

(HMSO, 1983). Szasz (2003) suggests that the use of statute to impose any form of treatment or intervention is open to individual interpretation and therefore abuse and reinforces the concept of psychiatry as a tool of social control. It is a matter of concern that skills that immobilise the hand by means of flexing wrist joints have the inadvertent corollary of impinging upon the fundamental right of freedom of expression when applied to a deaf service user. In view of the stance taken by the Human Rights Commission, what can be more inhumane or degrading than refusing a person their fundamental right to communicate their concerns about their treatment **at the time that such concern occurs**? This has potential implications for Article 10, which suggests that all individuals have the right to:

> Freedom of expression (HMSO, 1998, p. 31)

In view of this, skills used with deaf people should reflect the needs of all stakeholders, not least the deaf person who is being held. Guidelines exist that underpin the notion that methods used to manage aggressive behaviour should recognise the diversity of service users in our care (NICE, 2005; NIMHE, 2004; NASMHPD, 2002)

PROFESSIONAL CONTEXT AND DEAFNESS

Since professional codes are based upon the concept of beneficence, the decision to employ holding skills is a constant dilemma for care staff (Marangos-Frost and Wells, 2000). This involves the friction between intervening to protect self and others and the simultaneous duty of care to the service user's autonomy (Hinsby and Baker, 2004).

It is a point of note that legal frameworks often work towards the minimum standard of behaviour society expects from its citizens. The expectations of professional codes operate on **maximum** standards. This premise, to some degree, compounds the dilemma faced by carers when confronted with challenging behaviour that presents risk. On the one hand the law may consider interventions not in breach of statute, but professionally the carer may be criticised under the code from which they draw fundamental guidance.

Within generic mental health services, the use of restraint is often viewed by service users as evidence of the use of nurses to exercise power, enforce hospital rules and thus engage in coercive practice (Hopton, 1995). Since there has been little study in terms of the subjective restraint experiences of deaf service users, it can only be assumed that this would be a constant. What has been identified is that service users' and carers' perceptions of the event are different (Bonner *et al.*, 2002). There are different expectations placed upon both parties **by** both parties, and the upshot is inevitably a discourse of blame that perpetrates potential damage to the therapeutic alliance (Benson *et al.*, 2003). Anger and anxiety have been identified as two of the few elements of parity between staff and service users during and after the restraint process. Again this lack of congruence between the subjective experiences of staff and service users may have a negative impact upon future events.

In their study of staff responses to restraining service users, Sequeira and Halstead (2004) note that nurses involved in repeated incidents of restraint with the same person felt anger that they had been placed in a situation whereby they could find no alternative but to intervene at a physical level. This was particularly relevant to a diagnosis of personality disorder (PD) since staff would appear to be less tolerant and more reactionary over time to the behaviours of such individuals. This is a major concern considering reports that long-term exposure to the restraint process can create a sense of desensitisation in care staff that can promote jaded attitudes (Duxbury, 2002).

Service users' views of C&R were also studied by Sequeira and Halstead (2002). An emergent theme was that of how angry service users felt about the restraint experience. A predominant factor was that of the sense of injustice service users felt in the decision to use physical intervention. During the restraint process, service users have reported that they have been able to sense the carers' anger in the way that carers hold onto them. Given that touch is fundamental to a deaf person's communication, it is reasonable to suggest that the deaf service user will be more receptive to such dynamics if they should occur.

How care staff deal with the anxiety of managing challenging behaviour is also an area that is poorly researched. Some studies suggest that staff use humour to cope (Sequeira and Halstead, 2004). However, service users interpret humour during and post restraint as inappropriate and uncaring.

There is an argument that, while anger can be considered a constant within this process, respective loss of control is a possible pivotal element within the event dynamic. For the service user, loss of control means an assault upon their autonomy. For care staff, the need to ensure their legal and moral duty of care to the service user, their colleagues and themselves as individuals means potentially employing physical skills in an attempt to minimise all risk, and thus 'control' the environment.

CULTURAL COGENCE AND THERAPEUTIC HOLDING

An important question in the search for cultural cogence is 'What options do we leave the service user once their principal mode of communication has been removed?' There is a risk in an escalation in behaviour but also the potential of a further assault upon their dignity. If a deaf person is held in wrist locks or fixed mechanical restraints, they can only use their voice. Some deaf people find using their voice adds to their frustration and embarrassment. They may turn to aggressive behaviours to communicate these frustrations. By failing to acknowledge the limitations of existing methods of physical intervention, the deaf person's options narrow to the point where challenging behaviours may occur or at least perpetuate.

It has been identified that deaf people define their culture by the use of native sign language (Harris, 1995; Lane *et al.*, 1996). Cultural cogence is therefore enhanced by the active facilitation of sign language during the restraint process. A core belief in therapeutic holding is that managing movement is preferable to immobilisation (Stirling and McHugh, 1998). This process allows staff to work with the person as opposed to concentrating solely upon the presenting behaviour, allowing de-escalation skills to permeate into the crisis event, even when staff hold onto the service user (McHugh *et al.*, 1995). Therapeutic holding also facilitates the use of sign language.

There is consensus that communication needs to remain throughout any incident of restraint (NICE, 2005). If it is deemed that the presenting risk requires staff to use more restrictive methods of management, there may be methods used to facilitate communication that would leave the care staff and the service user being held less compromised. This is no less important when considering the physical impact of holding the deaf person. Injuries to the service user's hands will have long-term implications on their ability to communicate and may well serve as a daily reminder of the event in which it occurred. Justifiably, service users look at the physical after-effects of restraint with a sense of anger, which has clear implications for future relationships with the staff involved (Hopton, 1995; Whittington and Wykes, 1994). Damage to the therapeutic alliance post restraint can only be alleviated by proactive practice that underpins a notion of care over control (Duxbury and Whittington, 2005). Effectiveness of any physical intervention will be limited without the active promotion and investment in the therapeutic alliance (Duxbury, 2002).

If it is acknowledged that the dynamics of holding can effect the staff–patient/service user relationship, this must transfer to the use of interpreters during the crisis event. Once involved, they could be associated with the restraint post incident and damage their relationship with the service user. This is also relevant to good signing staff maintaining therapeutic relationships with the person. What can be argued here is that restraint that appropriately seeks to manage risk and maintain the safety of all stakeholders would be considered justified within legal, ethical and professional parameters if quality communication was established and maintained. Care staff who work with deaf people are therefore obligated to raise their standards of communication and immerse themselves within the cultural aspects of the people they aim to help.

This also leads to the role of deaf staff within the therapeutic holding process. There are clear communication issues when deaf staff hold onto the deaf person in crisis. Mehrabian (1981) suggests that communication is multifaceted and that non-verbal language remains a predominant factor during instances of anger and aggression. The use of touch is a powerful tool. Being held by a deaf peer is arguably no less threatening than being held by a hearing person, but may limit the sense of oppression felt by the deaf service user.

As we introduce the concept of deaf carers playing a pivotal role in the holding process, the practicalities of ongoing communication between hearing staff and their deaf contemporaries, plus the service user, become apparent. This is also an area that is in urgent need of attention since the effectiveness of the de-escalation process hinges upon maintaining a proactive dialogue. Practical issues have only been explored at a rudimentary level, and national consensus is required to address this fundamental issue (Anderson *et al.*, 2002). Figure 11.1 gives some examples of the multiplicities of communication that can be fostered and maintained before, during and after therapeutic holding.

The involvement of native sign language users enhances ongoing communication. Deaf staff involved in the therapeutic-holding process can identify subtle sign language nuances, clarify misconception and sharpen dialogue. In such highly charged events, there is no room for misconception and misunderstanding.

Proactive Practice	The Use of Touch	Facilitating Communication	Promoting Autonomy	Supportive Process
Establishing relationships Early intervention Care planning Risk assessment	No pain No flexing of wrists Appropriate levels of reassuring touch (comforting/ supporting) Least restrictive practice	Use of native sign language users Use of interpreters Developing good levels of BSL Deaf awareness	Advanced directives Service user involvement Least restrictive practice	Equitable support structure for service users and staff Post-incident debrief Subjective experience of event

Figure 11.1 Factors that facilitate effective communication before during and after therapeutic holding

These issues indicate a clear need for future research to focus upon the subjective experience of the deaf service user who has been restrained. There is a paucity of information within hearing mental health services, but in the realms of deaf people this aspect has not been explored in any great depth, if at all.

Cultural cogence cannot be attained without meaningful dialogue and mutual understanding. Collaborative approaches to working with aggressive service users are becoming the standard in UK mental health care (NIMHE, 2004). This needs to extend to deaf people in our care. Services working with deaf people will need to be aware of the principles of good practice when designing policies that manage challenging behaviour. Key factors in the UK hinge upon the inclusion of service users in policy design and service development (DoH, 1998). In aggression management, this extends to the provision of training, though in reality this is inconsistently applied. Where such philosophies have been embraced, a tangible reduction in violent incidents becomes an attainable ideal (Green and Robinson, 2005). This deficit must be overcome if cultural cogence is to ensue.

Using tools that promote collaborative practice, e.g. advanced directives, may provide the key to empowering deaf service users. Such demands are reinforced by service users themselves (Duxbury and Whittington, 2005). Using post-incident support can also generate a culture that serves to facilitate learning from each incident as opposed to merely reacting to the behaviour. Support must include both service user and staff in active discourse. Deaf staff may find themselves in a position whereby they have to hold onto a person they went to school with or someone they may know well from their Deaf Club. Support structures need to allow an opportunity for such matters to be raised and mooted constructively and effectively.

Educational programmes for all staff exposed to frequent episodes of challenging behaviour are vital to ensure such dynamics are given credence in practice. Deaf staff will require access to training packages that ultimately meet their explicit needs. This should include access to training in managing challenging behaviour using therapeutic-holding skills or non-aversive techniques that are not dependent upon the infliction of pain to be effective.Training programmes within specialist mental health services for deaf people should also deliver deaf awareness packages within any aggression-management courses; coupled with diversity and cultural competency.

CONCLUSION

The use of physical interventions within mental health care need to be consistently challenged considering the ethical, legal and professional tenets that question their imposition.

The introduction of C&R, usually synonymous with pain, has informed and shaped aggression-management delivery over the past twenty years. The author believes that such philosophies have no place in the management of deaf service users in crisis and can only compound issues of oppression, emasculation and cultural incongruity.

In using C&R with deaf service users, there is a risk that BSL is inhibited, leaving the deaf person no choice but to communicate through challenging behaviour. Therapeutic holding had been suggested as an alternative to active physical restraint since it encourages communication through touch and managing movement. This is vital with deaf service users, who need to move to communicate and rely on touch in a different way from a hearing person.

The use of native sign language users has been established as vital in the management of the deaf person in crisis. The need for greater levels of BSL in hearing care staff is another issue that must be addressed in any facility that provides care to deaf people with challenging behaviours. Without these key elements developing, cultural cogence will be made less effective and may bring care staff into conflict with ethical, legal and professional tenets each time they must intervene in a time of crisis.

REFERENCES

Anderson J, Eccles J, Harrington K, Horne N *et al.* (2002) *C&R Techniques and Deaf People: A Discussion Paper*, Bury, Mayflower Hospitals Ltd.

Beauchamp TL, Childress JF (2001) *Principles of Biomedical Ethics* (5th edn.), Oxford, Oxford University Press.

Beech B (2001) Managing aggression and violence in care settings: a review of the legal and ethical content of staff training courses. *Journal of Adult Protection* 3(9): 8–17.

Benson A, Secker J, Balfe E, Lipsedge M *et al.* (2003) Discourses of blame: accounting for aggression and violence on an acute mental health inpatient unit. *Social Science and Medicine* 57(5): 917–26.

Blofield J, Sallah D, Sashidaran S, Stone R, Struthers J (2003) *Independent Inquiry into the Death of David Bennett HSG (94) 27*, Cambridge, Norfollk, Suffolk and Cambridgeshire Strategic Health Authority Publication.

Bonner G, Lowe T, Rawcliffe D, Wellman N (2002) Trauma for all: a pilot study of the subjective experience of physical restraint for mental health inpatients and staff in the UK. *Journal of Psychiatric and Mental Health Nursing* 9(4): 465–73.

Citizens Commission on Human Rights (2004) *Deadly Restraints: Psychiatry's Therapeutic Assault: Report and Recommendations on Violent and Dangerous Use of Restraints in Mental Health Facilities*, Los Angeles, CCHR.

Colaizzi J (2005) Seclusion and restraint: a historical perspective. *Journal of Psychosocial Nursing* 43(2): 31–7.

Department of Health (1998) *A First Class Service: Quality in the New NHS*, London, TSO.

Duxbury J (2002) An evaluation of staff and patient views of and strategies employed to manage patient aggression and violence on one mental health unit: a pluralistic design. *Journal of Psychiatric and Mental Health Nursing* 9(3): 325–37.

Duxbury J, Whittington R (2005) Causes and management of patient aggression and violence: staff and patient perspectives. *Journal of Advanced Nursing* 50(5): 469–78.

Gournay K (2001) Violence in mental health care: are there any solutions? *Mental Health Practice* 5(2): 20–2.

Green B, Robinson L (2005) Reducing violence in a forensic mental health unit: a seven-year study. *Mental Health Practice* 9(4): 40–4.

Harris J (1995) *The Cultural Meaning of Deafness*. Aldershot, Ashgate.

Hinsby K, Baker M (2004) Patient and nurse accounts of violent incidents in a medium secure unit. *Journal of Psychiatric and Mental Health Nursing* 11(4): 341–7.

HMSO (1983) *Mental Health Act*, London, TSO.

HMSO (1998) *Human Rights Act*, London, TSO.

Hopton J (1995) Control and restraint in contemporary psychiatric nursing: some ethical considerations. *Journal of Advanced Nursing* 22(1): 110–15.

Jeffery D, Austen S (2005) Adapting de-escalation techniques with deaf service users. *Nursing Standard* 19(49): 41–7.

Kitson N, Fernando J, Douglas J (2000) Psychodynamic therapies: psychotherapy. In Hindley P, Kitson N (eds), *Mental Health and Deafness*, London, Whurr, pp. 337–56.

Lane H, Hoffmeister R, Bahan B (1996) *A Journey into the Deaf-World*, San Diego, Dawn Sign Press.

Marangos-Frost S, Wells D (2000) Psychiatric nurses' thoughts and feelings about restraint use: a decision dilemma. *Journal of Advanced Nursing* 31(2): 362–9.

McHugh A, Wain I, West M (1995) Handle with care. *Nursing Times* 91(6): 62–3.

Mehrabian A (1981) *Silent Messages: Implicit Communication of Emotions and Attitudes* (2nd edn.), Belmont, CA, Wadsworth.

National Association of State Mental Health Programme Directors (2002) *Reducing the Use of Seclusion and Restraint Part III: Lessons from the Deaf and Hard of Hearing Communities: A Technical Report*, Alexandra, VA, NASMHPD.

National Institute for Clinical Excellence (2005) *The Short-term Management of Disturbed/Violent Behaviour in In-patient Psychiatric Settings and Emergency Departments*, London, TSO.

National Institute for Mental Health in England (2004) *Developing Positive Practice to Support the Safe and Therapeutic Management of Aggression and Violence in Mental Health In-patient Settings: Mental Health Policy Implementation Guide*, London, Department of Health.

Paterson B (2005) Thinking the unthinkable: a role for pain compliance and mechanical restraint in the management of violence? *Mental Health Practice* 8(4): 18–23.

Ritchie S (1985) *Report to the Secretary of State for Social Services Concerning the Death of Mr Michael Martin*, London, SHSA.

Royal College of Psychiatrists (1998) *Management of Imminent Violence: Clinical Guidelines to Support Mental Health Services OP41*, London, Royal College of Psychiatrists.

Sequeira H, Halstead S (2002) Control and restraint in the UK: service user perspectives *The British Journal of Forensic Practice* 4(1): 9–18.

Sequeira H, Halstead S (2004) The psychological effects on nursing staff of administering physical restraint in a secure psychiatric hospital: 'When I go home, it's then that I think about it'. *The British Journal of Forensic Practice* 6(1): 3–15.

Smith SB (1995) Restraints: retraumatization for rape victims? *Journal of Psychosocial Nursing and Mental Health Services* 33(7): 23–8.

Stirling C, McHugh A (1998) Developing a non-aversive intervention strategy in the management of aggression and violence for people with learning disabilities using natural therapeutic holding. *Journal of Advanced Nursing* 27(3): 503–9.

Szasz TS (1989) *Law, Liberty and Psychiatry*, New York, Syracuse University Press.

Szasz TS (2003) *The Myth of Mental Illness: Foundations of a Theory of Personal Conduct* (rev. edn.), Revised Edition, New York, Perennial.

Tarbuck P (1992a) Use and abuse of control and restraint *Nursing Standard* 6(52): 30–2.

Tarbuck P (1992b) Ethical standards and human rights. *Nursing Standard* 7(6): 27–30.

United Kingdom Central Council (2002) *The Recognition, Prevention and Therapeutic Management of Violence in Mental Health Care: A Summary*, London, UKCC.

Watson R (2002) Assessing the need for restraint in older people. *Nursing Older People* 14(4): 31–2.

Whittington R, Wykes T (1994) Going in strong: confrontative coping by staff following assault by a patient. *Journal of Forensic Psychiatry* 5(3): 609–14.

12

A Model for Restraint Prevention in Residential Treatment for Deaf Children

JUDITH VREELAND

INTRODUCTION

The use of physical restraint in residential treatment facilities serving children with emotional and psychiatric disorders has come to be accepted as a necessary and appropriate intervention. Some have even suggested that it can have therapeutic value, communicating safety and containment to an out-of-control child (Ziegler, 2004). In the author's opinion the use of violent and traumatizing interventions should not be viewed as acceptable therapeutic tools. This chapter will challenge assumptions regarding the use of physical restraint and present a model for working toward the elimination of its use in residential treatment with deaf and hard-of-hearing children.

Walden School, a program of The Learning Center for Deaf Children in Framingham, Massachusetts, USA, is a residential school and treatment facility serving deaf and hard-of-hearing children with severe emotional, behavioral and psychiatric disabilities. The model presented in this chapter was developed by a project team representing all disciplines within the treatment facility and resulted in a 90% drop in the use of restraint over a four-year period.

Deafness and Challenging Behaviour: The 360° Perspective. Edited by S. Austen and D. Jeffery
© 2007 John Wiley & Sons Ltd

WHAT IS 'RESTRAINT'?

There are a number of ways in which treatment facilities intervene physically when a child is seriously self-abusive and/or assaultive.

- Physical restraint involves holding someone against his/her will.
- Mechanical restraint is the use of devices, such as straps, to secure an individual to a bed or stretcher.
- Chemical restraint is forced medication, usually in the form of an injection, to sedate an individual against his/her will.
- Seclusion is locked isolation and usually requires physically forcing a child into the room.

Walden School has never used mechanical or chemical restraints or seclusion. When the term 'restraint' is used in this chapter, it refers to physical restraint only. However, the concerns raised apply to all forms of restraint as well as seclusion.

BACKGROUND

THE CHALLENGE

Many children in residential treatment have long histories of neglect and abuse; some have lost their families, either through abandonment or the termination of parental rights. Children and youth who have suffered such trauma tend not, with good reason, to trust adults. Experience has taught them that adults are dangerous and will hurt children with their words, their fists or their groping hands. Because of these early experiences, children and youth with significant trauma histories often do not have the skills to accurately assess the safety of social situations. They may react to benign events with a level of fear or anger that seems out of proportion. Many of these children have also learned that the way to respond to feelings of anger, frustration or fear is through violence. In addition, no matter how painful or unsafe their homes may have been, these children still long for the family from whom they have been separated and may view staff in the treatment program as somehow responsible for, or as a painful reminder of, that loss. And so, treatment programs serving abused and abandoned children are faced with the challenge of caring for children who are experiencing intense rage, fear and despair, and for whom the learned response to these feelings is violence. It is the responsibility of those who serve these children to give them reason to trust that not all adults will hurt them and to help them develop strategies other than violence to protect themselves and deal with the rage they carry within them. Often, current practices fail to meet these challenges.

CONTROL VERSUS TREATMENT

Though exceptions exist, standard practice in the field often operates on the assumption that children need to be contained, controlled and directed (Fox, 1994). Many residential treatment programs employ elaborate and artificial systems of points and levels, turning much needed activities and community experiences into privileges to be earned. The goal becomes forced compliance rather than healing and growth.

> Having points and level systems which apply equally to all children/youth in a program is the same as giving identical medical treatment to all patients, regardless of their diagnosis. How is it 'fair' to expect the same of all children, when those in the program come to us, in fact, with a very wide variety of issues and problems? (Fox, 1994, p. 17)

In many programs, numerous non-negotiable rules are often established by the adults in power and enforced with little room for discussion. When this leads, as it inevitably does, to a power struggle, the escalating incident often ends with the child resorting to physical aggression.

The standard treatment program approach to addressing this dilemma is to train staff in how to physically restrain aggressive children and youth. There are many packaged training programs that certify staff in what is called 'non-violent physical intervention'. People are trained how to hold a violent individual in a manner that is designed to minimize the risk of injury to all involved. These training programs also teach interventions designed to de-escalate the situation and reduce the need for restraint, and they strongly emphasize that physical restraint should be the absolute last option after all other intervention strategies have failed. Some training programs, such as the one in use at Walden School, also stress that restraint is dangerous and can result in serious injury or death. The intent is to be certain staff take restraint very seriously and do all they possibly can do to avoid restraining a child.

In theory, this approach seems reasonable as a way to safely manage aggressive children. In practice, however, in our experience it often creates an environment that is counter to the treatment needs of these children and youth. The reality is that the experience of physical restraint re-traumatizes the child and reinforces his/her belief that adults will physically force children to do things (Fox, 2004). Restraint does not promote healing; it communicates the acceptance of physical force as a means of obtaining compliance. And it is not safe. It is estimated that 50 to 150 deaths occur in the USA each year as a result of seclusion and restraint (Bullard *et al.*, 2003). The problem is further compounded by the lack of professional training and experience of most staff working in treatment programs. Because salaries are low, the work extremely difficult, the hours undesirable and societal recognition virtually nonexistent, those entrusted with the care of these vulnerable children usually come to their positions with no experience or formal training to do this work (Drais-Parrillo, 2003). Learning to engage with these children in ways that earn their trust and can help them find new ways to manage intense emotions is extremely difficult and requires a great deal of practice. It requires a sophisticated understanding of child development and the psychological impact of childhood trauma. By contrast, traditional approaches to discipline – limit setting, followed by demand, followed by punishment for non-compliance – are much easier for the novice child care worker. This is also, however, the approach that will often intensify a traumatized child's anger. And so a negative pattern emerges (Figure 12.1). Staff set a limit. The child does not comply. The limit is repeated more sternly. The child becomes more defiant. A power struggle ensues, and it eventually leads to restraint. Practice shows that, when restraint is offered as an intervention, its need is assumed and it becomes far too commonplace unless the treatment model, supported by clear policies and procedures, offers other tools to staff, and intensive training and supervision are in place to help staff learn effective strategies (Kirkland, 2003).

CHANGE PROCESS

REFRAMING RESTRAINT

The first step in reducing the use of physical restraint and moving toward its elimination is to reframe the use of restraint from a treatment intervention to an indication of a treatment failure. It must be

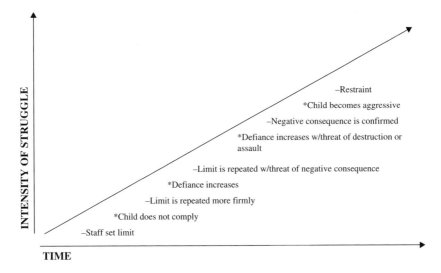

Figure 12.1 Power struggle leading to restraint

emphasized, however, that by this we mean a failure of the system, of the treatment plan and strategies and **not** the individuals working directly with the child. The intent is not to blame individuals but to create a culture in which physical restraint can never be viewed as a therapeutic intervention. While a restraint system may claim to be non-violent, in our observations a child being restrained experiences the event as an act of violence. When a restraint is initiated, the child typically becomes more enraged and struggles with those who are holding him/her. The more the child struggles, the more staff struggle to maintain control. The child may be held against a wall, or moved face down to the floor, a position that can cause frightening flashbacks for the child with a sexual abuse history. The experience for the child is far too familiar. Adults grab you, pin you down and render you powerless.

Acknowledging that restraint is antitherapeutic does not suggest that children who have become dangerously assaultive or are poised to run into traffic should be permitted to harm themselves or others. Clearly, at this point, blocking, and perhaps physically restraining, the child is necessary. The **need** for restraint, however, is what constitutes the treatment failure. How did the child get to this point and what might have been done earlier to prevent such escalation?

EFFECTIVE RESTRAINT-REDUCTION PROGRAMS

Through on-site visits and ongoing conversations with professionals at other schools and agencies with successful restraint-reduction projects, as well as our own experiences implementing changes within Walden School, it became clear that effective restraint-reduction programs had elements in common. These common program components included:

- an emphasis, in policy and practice, on the dangers of restraint
- shared commitment/shared leadership
- a system of accountability
- a strength-based treatment model that emphasizes relationship building and the development of social skills
- inclusion of children and families in the treatment process
- a comprehensive staff-training curriculum.

An Emphasis, in Policy and Practice, on the Dangers of Restraint

Emphasizing the danger of restraint in the context of crisis-intervention training is only the beginning. This must be reflected in written policy and acknowledged in all discussions of intervention strategies with potentially assaultive or self-abusive children. When a child is restrained, the discussion of what went wrong must focus on issues of programming and service delivery, not the child's inappropriate actions or failure to comply. It is already known that the child has difficulty regulating his/her emotions and has come to the facility for help. When there is a treatment failure resulting in restraint, it is the responsibility of the professionals to examine their actions and make changes in programming and interventions as they continue to seek ways to help the child heal and grow.

Shared Commitment/Shared Leadership

To be effective, the effort to reduce/eliminate the use of restraint must be an agency-wide commitment to which all staff have the opportunity to have meaningful input and decision-making authority. Full support of the agency leaders is essential, but it cannot be a top-down dictate (Masker and Steele, 2004).

As members of the Walden School community began to perceive the use of restraint as a dangerous impediment to treatment, a widespread commitment to work toward change emerged. That commitment led to the establishment of a project team to organize and lead the change process. Participation was open to all and membership was determined through self-selection. The only requirements were that those who join believe in the goal of eliminating restraints (even if they had questions about if or how it could be accomplished), expected to stay with the agency for at least a year and were willing to commit to attending meetings and doing additional work. Fifteen volunteers came forward, more than half of them direct service providers, and all departments were represented.

When restraint is no longer assumed to be an acceptable intervention and is instead considered a treatment failure, it becomes apparent that working toward its elimination involves all aspects of programming, from philosophy to practice. The project team met monthly and broke into working committees that met more frequently to conduct research and make recommendations. The areas addressed by committees included programming, policies and procedures, staff training, facilities, youth involvement and family involvement.

A System of Accountability

Debriefings

If a child is restrained at Walden School, a three-page incident report is written by the primary staff person engaged with the child and signed by all staff involved in any way. The report is reviewed by the assistant director, who is also the lead crisis-intervention trainer. Questions or concerns are noted, and the report then goes to the supervisor of the reporting staff. All staff in all positions at Walden School receive weekly individual supervision that provides support, offers guidance and feedback and reviews interventions to maximize safety. In this context, the written report will then be reviewed with the employee. A debriefing is scheduled with all staff involved and, in most instances, the child who was restrained. The purpose of the debriefing is to examine what led to the need for restraint, and what could have been done differently to prevent the escalation. The program must be held accountable for treatment failures, and individuals must accept responsibility for mistakes, but the intent of debriefings is to learn through open examination. It is not a disciplinary meeting.

Goal-setting and Data Reviews

Setting specific goals for restraint reduction keeps the issue a high priority and helps motivate members of the treatment community (Bullard *et al.*, 2003). Walden School also celebrates significant milestones on the quest toward eliminating restraints, hosting late-afternoon parties with the children and staff in which a visual presentation of the achievement is unveiled and later displayed in the hall as they continue to work toward the next goal.

Careful data collection and review offer another means of accountability. Walden School produces monthly charts tracking the incident reports written on each child. Such reports are written each time a serious incident occurs. This includes, but would not be limited to, incidents resulting in the use of physical restraint. These charts show breakdowns by days of the week, time of day and type of incident. They allow supervisors and staff to look for patterns that might be useful in developing appropriate programming and intervention strategies. The charts can also be reviewed with youth to help them better understand their behavior and explore coping strategies. Program data are also reviewed and collected on a monthly basis, and restraint numbers are reported back to staff.

Surveys and Interviews

Staff surveys and student interviews provided additional data on how restraint was used and perceived by members of the Walden School community, and led to further discussion of the hopes and concerns raised by a commitment to end the use of restraint as an intervention. The surveys were completed at unit and department meetings to maximize participation. More importantly, completing the surveys in this way helped reduce the language barriers that may arise when English is a second language for many staff. Roughly 70% of employees at Walden School are deaf and identify American Sign Language (ASL) as their primary language. By completing the surveys in the meetings, questions could be presented in ASL and employees could, and did, turn to one another for additional clarification as needed before writing their responses.

Face-to-face interviews were conducted periodically with students to learn more about how they experienced restraint, to keep them involved in the process and to obtain their views on the progress of the project.

A Strength-based Treatment Model that Emphasizes Relationship Building and the Development of Social Skills

Walden School's treatment model was significantly changed as a result of the work of the project team. The model was developed using the Circle of Courage, a Native American concept of youth development built upon the belief that children must always be treated with respect and dignity.

> Native American philosophies of child management represent what is perhaps the most effective system of positive discipline ever developed. These approaches emerged from cultures where the central purpose of life was the education and empowerment of children ... We propose belonging, mastery, independence, and generosity as the central values – the unifying themes – of positive cultures for education and youth work programs. (Brendtro *et al.*, 2002, p. 45)

Walden School has used this circle as the foundation for its program of healing and growth. This program provides a structure in which to identify strengths and needs and establish goals in the context of the four core values: belonging, generosity, mastery and independence.

The Walden School Circle of Courage program defines treatment as a path of self-exploration and personal growth, and stages within the program help structure the work being done by the child and his/her team. These stages should not be perceived as program levels. They are not linked with privileges, nor are they earned or lost based on compliance. Rather, the Circle of Courage program is a treatment curriculum. Each stage offers guidelines and activities that enable residential, educational and clinical staff to work together with the child and their family to identify and achieve personal goals. The program is designed to build upon existing strengths, foster a sense of community, provide opportunities to develop and practise new skills and to formally celebrate progress.

Programming also focuses on the creation of services and activities that help children develop relationship skills and coping strategies. These include community-service projects on and off campus, welcoming ceremonies for new students, monthly social events planned by student/staff teams, a relaxation room offering sensory integration and stress-reduction activities, a community garden and a weekly yoga class.

To effectively implement a treatment model based on the development relationships and social skills, staff must share a common language with the children and have an understanding and respect for their culture. Cultural and linguistic competence have been identified as factors in restraint reduction.

> Staff members must be sensitive to cultural differences. Staff members should be able to recognize phrases, tones, volume, cadence, and physical gestures and postures that might be misinterpreted by a child and thus provoke behavior crises. In addition, staff members must be able to provide information to the child and family members in a linguistically and developmentally appropriate manner. (Bullard *et al.*, 2003, p. 15)

All of the children served at Walden School are deaf or hard of hearing and use ASL as their primary language. Significantly more than half of those working at Walden School are also deaf. Those who are not, with the exception of a few support staff such as a part-time nurse or cook, possess a second-language fluency in ASL. To benefit from milieu treatment, a deaf child must be in an environment that is fully accessible. He/she must be able to communicate freely and directly with peers, caretakers, teachers, therapists, supervisors and administrators.

Inclusion of Children and Families in the Treatment Process

Reducing the use of physical restraint requires working as partners with children and their families. At Walden School, the child is an active participant in the Circle of Courage program, meeting with his/her team periodically to develop, review and revise a skill-building plan. This plan includes three parts: identification of strengths, goal-setting relevant to the four core values and strategies for identifying and managing intense emotional reactions. Walden School also has a youth leadership council that creates a forum in which residents have meaningful input into program policies and procedures.

Inclusion of families is particularly challenging for programs serving deaf children and youth because the geographic region served tends to be much larger than the typical treatment program serving hearing children. Though located in Massachusetts, Walden School has served children and families from up and down the east coast of the United States, and in some instances the midwest and western part of the country. When a new child is entering the program, the parents or guardians are interviewed to obtain their views of the child's strengths and needs in nine life domains. The admission plan will be developed with the family, and for out-of-state families may include a period of time in which the family stays on campus to assist with the transition. This helps the child adjust to the move and allows the family to become familiar with the people to whom they are entrusting the care of their child. Walden School has a house on campus that is designated as the family residence, and families stay there free of charge. This is invaluable not only during the admissions process but for ongoing family visits and therapy sessions as well.

All families have weekly contact with a therapist in the program. If they are unable to be physically present for treatment-planning meetings, they are invited to attend by phone conference or, if that is not possible, their input is obtained by the therapist prior to the meeting.

All family members now also receive a newsletter specifically detailing the work of the project team and the programming changes implemented as a part of that work.

A Comprehensive Staff-training Curriculum

Traditionally, one of the first and most extensive courses offered to new staff in a treatment program is crisis intervention, including the use of physical restraint. This tends to be followed quickly by other trainings mandated by licensing agencies such as First Aid, Reporting Suspected Abuse and Neglect, Medication Education, and Emergency Procedures. While all are clearly important, as an initial training cluster, they communicate risk, pathology and criminal behavior. This emphasis runs counter to the concepts of strength-based programming.

With staff working multiple shifts covering seven days a week, 24 hours a day, the scheduling of staff training presents a huge challenge, but it is a challenge that must be met. Most direct care staff come to their jobs with little or no experience or formal training to work with challenging children and youth. Evidence has shown that training focused on positive milieu treatment, including understanding the population served, relationship building, active listening, avoiding power struggles and conflict management is linked to a significant reduction in the use of restraint (Bullard et al., 2003). It is, therefore, essential to create a training curriculum that offers new staff a series of workshops and classes that frame their work as caregivers and teachers, and gives them the skills to do the job.

Walden School developed a staff-training curriculum that began with introductory workshops designed to explain the principles of strength-based treatment and begin developing the skills to work effectively in a therapeutic milieu. Monthly workshops are then offered on a rotating basis to further develop skills and address specific aspects of treatment, such as teaching generosity through community service or responding to sexualized behaviors in the milieu.

Case Study

Ray is a thirteen-year-old boy with a history of neglect and multiple traumas. He came to Walden School when he was nine, after the foster family that had planned to adopt him asked the state to remove him from their home. After repeated destructive and assaultive incidents, they felt they could not continue to care for him. He was hospitalized and diagnosed with attachment disorder and posttraumatic stress disorder. He was then moved directly from the hospital to Walden School. At the end of his first week in Walden School, the social worker from the state agency came to visit and informed him he would not be returning to the family with whom he had lived since he was six years old.

During Ray's first two years at Walden School, we saw a continuation of the behaviors he had displayed in foster care. Treatment plans were developed and goals set by the professionals. The clinical psychologist completed an evaluation and consulted with staff. Ray's individual therapist met with him two to three times a week. The educational and residential teams met regularly to identify problems and share strategies. Still, we did not see consistent progress, and concerns grew as each step forward seemed to be followed by two steps back. Ray was being physically restrained three to four times a month and was re-hospitalized five times during those first two years.

The changes initiated at Walden School as part of the project to reduce/eliminate restraints began to be implemented toward the end of Ray's second year in the program. When charts of his critical incidents were reviewed, several patterns emerged. For example, weekday mornings, before school, were clearly particularly difficult times. Previous to this project, discussion might have focused on what Ray needed to do differently in the morning; now staff were exploring what they might do differently to teach him how to better manage the morning transitions. The charts were shared with Ray, and he was engaged in discussions to determine why this was happening and how it could be addressed. From these discussions, a further pattern emerged.

Ray almost always woke up very early, prior to any other resident, and at least an hour and a half before breakfast was served. He tended to stay in his room, awake, thinking about school and growing increasingly anxious. By the time he came out of his room, he was often already agitated, though with no explanation. He was also usually quite hungry. He would tell staff he was hungry, only to be reminded of the time breakfast was served. He might then start pacing, teasing staff with sarcastic comments or physical pokes, or pushing limits, demanding staff attention in negative ways. As others began to wake up, he would shift his verbal and physical jabs to peers. These situations would then often escalate to serious struggles, which at times would lead to assaultive behavior and physical restraint.

Once the above pattern was more fully understood, Ray and his team were able to discuss how to make mornings more pleasant for everyone involved. Ray agreed to let staff know as soon as he was awake so that he would not start each day focused on his school anxieties. Staff offered to begin checking on him at 5.30 each morning, in case he was awake but having difficulty getting up. Fruit and breakfast bars were kept in the staff office so that if he was hungry before breakfast he could eat. Ray then identified activities that he enjoyed and might be able to do during the early morning to occupy his time in a pleasurable way. He went shopping with staff to purchase art materials and craft projects, as well as a couple of board games. A review of monthly incident charts for the three months following the implementation of these changes showed a dramatic reduction in early-morning incidents. This accomplishment was shared with others and celebrated at a community meeting.

Ray also attended meetings and worked with his team to develop a skill-building plan to identify strengths, triggers and coping strategies and set goals relevant to the four core values of the Circle of Courage. These meetings include the child, his therapist and two advocates, one from school, one from the residence. They are held in a private, comfortable office and beverages and snacks are served using special place settings reserved for these meetings only.

Identifying strengths is often one of the most difficult tasks for the child. They have been so often reminded of their failures and shortcomings that they have come to define themselves by what they lack or have not done well. Therefore, these meetings begin with and often devote considerable time to the identification of strengths. The form used offers many examples, ranging from concrete activities ('I can make things with my hands') to issues of self-care and appearance ('I take care of my body', 'I care about how I look') to relational strengths ('I enjoy making people laugh', 'I have friends who care about me'). Once Ray, with encouragement from staff, was able to identify strengths from the list, he began to elaborate and add new items ('I can make things with my hands – like big Lego buildings', 'I know a lot about my home state and can teach people about it').

Identifying the things that upset him was easier for Ray, but he took the discussion seriously and gained insights through this process. He also found it very helpful to talk with staff about early warning signs that he was becoming upset. He reported that when he said he was 'bored', he usually really meant he was becoming frustrated or angry, but it was more difficult for him to admit to those feelings. Ray was surprised to learn from staff that he often cracked his knuckles when he seems tense, but, once that was shared with him, he was able to catch himself doing it and learned to recognize it as an indication of mounting tensions or frustrations.

Discussion of triggers and warning signs leads naturally into the identification of coping strategies. Ray was able to identify numerous interventions that helped him calm down, some involving activities, such as dribbling a basketball, some relational (going for a walk with a favorite member of staff), and still others more solitary (practicing yoga).

All of the information arising from these discussions was then used to develop goals and objectives that truly meant something to the child. Ray's goals were his. Staff guided and supported him through the process, but he identified his strengths and his needs, and he was the creator of his goals.

Ray is now doing well. He remains at Walden School, but a foster family is actively being sought. He has not been hospitalized in over a year and has been restraint-free for six months.

RESULTS

Four years after the creation of the project team at Walden School, restraint usage has dropped by 90%. Nine of the original fifteen members are still actively involved, and six others have joined. We are continuing to develop policies and procedures that we hope will move us closer to our goal of eliminating the need for restraint, particularly in the areas of new staff orientation and training practices and greater inclusion of children and family members in all aspects of service delivery.

CONCLUSION

To reduce and eliminate the need for physical restraint in residential treatment requires an organized and comprehensive approach that is truly about much more than restraint. It begins with a clear definition of restraint as antitherapeutic. The agency must then make a commitment to openly challenge beliefs and practices, to include the entire community in the change effort, to establish a clear system of accountability and to develop a relationship-based treatment model.

REFERENCES

Brendtro L, Brokenleg M, Van Bockern S (2002) *Reclaiming Youth At Risk*, Bloomington, IN, National Education Service.

Bullard L, Fulmore D, Johnson K (2003) *Reducing the Use of Restraint and Seclusion*, Washington, CWLA Press.

Drais-Parrillo A (2003) *Child Welfare League of America 2003 Salary Study*, Washington, CWLA Press.

Fox L (1994) The catastrophe of compliance. *The Journal of Child and Youth Care* 9(1): 13–22.

Fox L (2004) The impact of restraint on sexually abused children and youth. *Residential Group Care Quarterly* 4(3): 1–5.

Kirkland S (2003) Practicing restraint. *Children's Voices* 12(5): 14–19.

Masker A, Steele J (2004) Reducing physical management and time out: a five-year update on one agency's experience. *Residential Group Care Quarterly* 4(3): 6–7.

Ziegler D (2004) The therapeutic value of using physical interventions to address violent behavior in children, http://rccp.cornell.edu/pdfs/Zeigler1.pdf, accessed 28 June 2006.

13

The Role of Deaf Staff and Interpreters in Preventing Challenging Behaviour

ADRIAN HARPER AND MARY CONNELL

INTRODUCTION

Differences between hearing and Deaf culture, reliance on written material and an overdependence on oral means of communication can often leave the Deaf patient feeling disrespected, disempowered and uninformed. In this chapter, the authors argue that challenging behaviour can be prevented or reduced by the provision of a truly accessible environment for Deaf patients. It is argued that the absence of Deaf staff will result in increased challenging behaviour, endangering both the interpreter and the patient. The challenge of interpreting material that is highly charged is discussed and the role of the interpreter during physical restraint is described.

In order to prevent challenging behaviour, it is crucial that all staff are aware of their linguistic limitations and can take feedback from others as to how their language behaviour may be affecting patients. In this chapter, we draw from our experience of Deaf mental health services; however, much could be generalised to prisons, education settings or housing provision.

Deafness and Challenging Behaviour: The 360° Perspective. Edited by S. Austen and D. Jeffery
© 2007 John Wiley & Sons Ltd

ACCESSIBLE ENVIRONMENTS CAN REDUCE CHALLENGING BEHAVIOUR

This paper was written as a result of the authors' discussions with experienced Deaf staff about their work practices and includes Deaf perspectives on why patients sometimes become frustrated and why situations escalate into challenging behaviour. These Deaf staff reported that repeated cultural and linguistic mismatches are seen as disrespectful and are a common cause of frustration among patients.

THE IMPORTANCE OF DEAF STAFF

Deaf people in a hearing world often lack access to conversation and information and are therefore socially excluded. The resulting social isolation and low self-worth increase their vulnerability to mental ill-health (Ridgeway, 1997; Steinberg *et al.*, 1998; Du Feu and Fergusson, 2003). Ironically, this can even happen when the Deaf person is supposedly being treated in a mental health provision. Thus, in order to increase mental well-being, it seems logical to offer a positive model of social interaction with Deaf role models and the fluent signing environment as the foundation.

Respect towards Deaf patients' language and culture is an essential part of an effective Deaf mental health service. This may seem obvious but it remains the case that Deaf mental health services are mostly provided by hearing people. The authors would argue that Deaf staff can give a more linguistically and culturally appropriate service and in doing so they reduce the potential for challenging behaviour. Kitson and Klein (2000) report crucial gains from the systematic employment of Deaf mental health workers who can more readily understand patients, are more likely to be familiar with a variety of regional and social dialects and who, sharing the visual perspective, are able to frame information in a more accessible way.

Deaf people do not have equal access to education and training, and progress in training Deaf nurses has been slow (Kitson and Austen, 2004). It is likely that Deaf staff may make up only a small proportion of the workforce and/or be disproportionately employed in the lower-status roles (Watson *et al.*, 2005). Deaf staff are often underused but are a scarce and essential resource, and it may be necessary to view those with finely honed sign language skills and cultural know-how as possessing a qualification and to reward accordingly. A proactive recruitment of Deaf staff is required at all levels with adequate financial incentives and opportunities for professional training.

MAXIMISING DEAF/HEARING INTERACTION

Although the interpreter, Deaf relay interpreter and Deaf staff have crucial roles within mental health services, this should not detract from the need for hearing staff to maximise their own signing ability. Staff with less signing skills do not confidently share patients' space unless obliged to, for example when formally observing patients for safety reasons, or for their own benefit such as when watching TV in the patients' day room. This reduces opportunities for communication, which would be beneficial to both parties. For patients, interaction with staff can give them a sense of worth and open up chances for them to glean information; for staff it can increase their cultural knowledge as well as provide opportunities for monitoring the patients' mental health. Despite good intentions, hearing staff do sometimes forget to sign or sign whilst speaking, which reduces the quality of their signing.

Proactive Ways to Include Patients

- In a mental health inpatient setting, interpreters could assist hearing staff and Deaf patients to interact socially.
- Where staff are speaking, rather than signing, other staff or patients would ideally feel able to remind them to sign.
- Signing members of staff can proactively offer patients an opportunity to be included in conversations, for example summarising the ongoing conversation so they can choose to join in, 'We have been talking about such and such . . .'
- TV programs that have in-vision signing or are presented in sign language provide shared relaxation and stimulation for Deaf patients and hearing staff, as well as providing a focus for discussion and information-giving.
- Adopting national strategies that support service users' involvement at an operational and organisational level (Department of Health, 2000).

ACCESS TO INFORMATION: THE CURSE OF WRITTEN MATERIAL

Bibliotherapy is a common feature of modern mental health provision (Gregory *et al.*, 2004). However, literacy problems within the profoundly Deaf population (Conrad, 1979) can make the experience of inaccessible written material frustrating and demoralising and could lead to challenging behaviour. Embarrassed by their poor reading, or wanting to please the clinician, patients sometimes pretend to understand written text, which can lead to misunderstandings at a later date. Where possible, all written material should be translated into sign language or at the very least presented in plain English with ample illustrations.

RESPECTING DEAF PATIENTS AND THEIR CULTURE

Between any two cultures, misunderstandings are possible and behaviour that is experienced as disrespectful can give rise to hostility. There are some marked differences between hearing and Deaf culture.

- If hearing staff talk or laugh with each other, when sharing a space with patients, the excluded patient may think they are being talked about. This can lead to feelings of suspicion, which could arouse hostile feelings.
- Deaf staff greet each patient on meeting them and acknowledge their presence at appropriate junctures. Hearing staff unfamiliar with Deaf culture may feel self-conscious doing this. Deaf patients appreciate recognition through eye contact, and a wave or thumbs-up with a nod of acknowledgement speaks volumes.
- Hearing staff and Deaf patients may view the same situation differently. Hearing staff may not want to inflict their poor signing on the Deaf person or may inadvertently show their frustration at their own inability to communicate, e.g. by raising eyes to heaven or sighing. However, the visually astute Deaf patient may construe this as impatience and 'poor attitude'.
- Hearing culture relies on hints and subtleties at times of social embarrassment, whereas Deaf culture allows far more direct communication. However, Deaf staff report examples of hearing staff attempting to emulate this directness but omitting subtle facial and manual markers which modify the sign to indicate politeness, e.g. a

hearing nurse signing directly to a patient 'You smell and need a bath' but missing out the subtle non-manual features which a Deaf member of staff would have used with the effect of preceding this statement with 'I am really sorry to have to say this but . . .'

Hearing staff at all levels must receive intensive training in sign language and ongoing regular information on Deaf culture, Deaf awareness and Deaf issues. In areas with rapid staff turnover, temporary staff and staff working shifts, regular and creative sign language training is required.

THE ROLE OF DEAF STAFF IN MAXIMISING UNDERSTANDING

MONITORING THE SIGNING ABILITY OF HEARING STAFF

In the ideal Deaf mental health service all hearing staff would sign so well that they did not need interpreters. However, knowing the point at which one is competent to sign for oneself is a decision that the authors believe hearing staff should not make alone. Deaf staff should be involved in this decision by sitting in on sessions to help check the competency of hearing staff. Different patients require different levels of signing competency, and for staff to reach a level of fluency to enable them to sign for themselves is likely to involve a series of decisions within an ongoing process rather than a one-off 'graduation day'.

A culture of defensiveness or arrogance about signing skills is likely to fuel rather than prevent challenging behaviour. It is imperative that there is a working culture in which staff feel comfortable to intervene when they see another staff member involved in a miscommunication or potential miscommunication.

Case Study One

Patient: When are we going to the coffee shop? *(signing coffee shop as 'over there')*
Hearing staff: *(not fully understanding but pretending to)* Yes, we are going over there.
Patient: But **when** are we going? *(pointing at the clock on the wall)*

Hearing staff: *(not realising that patient is pointing at clock but still thinking he is gesturing about the direction of the coffee shop)* Yes, that's right, over there.

Patient: *(getting frustrated)* But **when**?

Hearing staff: *(getting frustrated at what they see as repeated questioning and not noticing the patient's body language)* Yes, that's right. We **are** going over there.

(The patient now feels ignored and is getting dangerously cross. A Deaf staff member steps in.)

USING VISUAL CONCEPTS

Working in a bilingual signing mental health environment requires more than just learning a second language. Patients are likely to have varying degrees of language ability either as a result of language deprivation and learning disability or as a result of their mental state as influenced by such things as schizophrenia, depression or anxiety. Good communication requires being able to conceptualise visually, a skill that Deaf staff have usually been honing since they were born. Whenever a patient is struggling to understand or is refusing to cooperate, it is important to check whether the explanation has in fact been given in a sufficiently visual form. The degree of visual representation required is inversely proportionally to the language skills and mental health of the patient.

Case Study Two

Patient X was refusing his medication and saying with increasing determination that the medication was wrong and would not help him. Senior (hearing) staff regarded the refusal as evidence of the patient's recalcitrance. A Deaf member of staff was involved and translated the dialogues into a pictorial form. As a result the cause of the patient's reluctance was discovered. The patient had been familiar with, and had put his trust in, a tablet of a particular colour. As the patient's mental health improved, he was prescribed a lower dose of his medication, which came in a different colour tablet. The patient was concerned that he was being offered a completely different and perhaps wrong medication.

The Role of the Mental Health Interpreter

An interpreter is someone who is (at least) bilingual but also has the ability and training to be able to work between two languages and facilitate communication between people. Many Deaf and hearing staff regularly interpret small amounts of information informally, but a professional interpreter requires a degree-level qualification. An interpreter working in a mental health setting requires not only a high level of fluency in sign language and spoken language but also knowledge and experience of mental health matters and should be able to function adequately with patients who are not straightforward users of sign language. Hamerdinger and Karlin (2003) question whether most interpreters are adequately trained for providing access to mental health services.

Bad interpreting disables rather than enables. In the absence of sufficient training or experience, the interpreter may make mistakes, which prevents the clinician from achieving the correct diagnosis and formulating the appropriate treatment plan. In a client group who may be prone to challenging behaviour, such mistakes could result in existing challenging behaviour being poorly treated or new episodes occurring iatrogenically.

Marcos (1979) expresses concern about standards of interpreting in mental health settings. In his opinion, interpreters need to be trained to self-monitor the tendency to 'filter' information, which may result in potentially distorting it in clinically significant ways. Interpreters, by the very nature of their role, are virtually programmed to make sense of language. In situations where the source language does not make sense as a result of the patient's condition, such as thought disorder or psychosis, there is a risk of the interpreter filtering and reproducing language that does make 'sense' and thereby distorts the message.

Napier and Cornes (2004) suggest cautiously switching between free and literal methods within an interpretation. Free interpretation espouses a holistic interpretation where interpreters endeavour to make sense of an utterance rather than providing word-for-sign (or sign-for-word) interpretations. A more literal approach may be more appropriate when utterances do not make sense or when a therapist needs to hear the stream of consciousness. Taylor (2002) cautions against culturally adjusting the language of the patient to present equivalent meaning without guidance from the clinician as to which information is relevant. Others sources of distortion identified by Marcos (1979) are deficient linguistic or interpreter skill, lack of knowledge and sophistication in mental health, and the interpreter's attitudes towards either patients or clinicians.

Given that the standard of interpreters varies, it is important to consider the clinical team's procedures for their booking. This responsibility often falls to hearing or administrative staff, thus failing to make use of the opinions and preferences of those with clinical experience and who are Deaf. In the authors' opinion, the advice of Deaf staff should be sought as to which interpreters are suitable and whether a Deaf relay interpreter should be used in situations where the interpreter is less experienced or the patient's presentation more complex.

DEAF RELAY INTERPRETERS

The role of Deaf relay interpreters (also referred to as intermediaries or Deaf interpreters) is being increasingly recognised, particularly in mental health.

> Some clients may use a non-standard form of sign language, which could be a result of their mental ill health and/or socio-linguistic factors. They may have a language disorder, visual difficulties, communication problems, or use sign languages other than BSL. For these clients it is useful to have a Deaf interpreter. (ASLI, 2005)

The Deaf interpreter relays the message from a sign language interpreter or hearing professional to the patient and vice versa. In relay interpreting, the Deaf interpreter will use their native signing skills and experience of 'code-switching' (switching between different modes and levels of sophistication of the same language) to enrich the clarity of the information. While there are many talented hearing interpreters, the relay interpreter has the advantage of years of experience of moving between, for example, British Sign Language, Sign Supported English, and mime and gesture, depending on the skills of the person with whom they are communicating (who could be deaf, Deaf or hearing).

Case Study Three

Mr Y was a native sign language user with severe premeditated and explosive challenging behaviour, who had been paralysed down one side by a stroke. To a non-native signer, his one-handed sign language resembled fairly basic gesture. Hearing stroke physicians assessed Mr Y using hearing interpreters and concluded that he had limited cognitive and linguistic abilities. A further assessment by a Deaf mental health team of his cognitive abilities was requested. During this assessment and with the help of a relay interpreter, Mr Y was seen to have above-average cognitive and linguistic skills. Such information was crucial in planning subsequent behaviour modification and in reducing the patient's communication frustration. Movements that the hearing interpreter had perceived as non-linguistic jerks and swinging of the arms the relay interpreter had understood as signs that were poorly executed as a result of his stroke damage. In an equivalent hearing patient, this would be similar to a non-native-English-speaking clinician trying to assess a stroke patient that slurred or mispronounced words compared to a flexible-native-English speaker assessing the same speech.

Deaf relay interpreters are also irreplaceable in the area of sign vocabulary development. In subject areas where there has previously been little involvement of Deaf professionals, sign language may have yet to fully develop to cover the sophisticated concepts, terminology and jargon used, to allow Deaf people equal access. The role of the Deaf interpreter can be particularly valuable in working with clinicians and hearing interpreters to develop signs and sign usage. For example, the development of consistent signs for different types of medication, symptoms and interventions reduces the need for finger spelling of complicated words. Similarly, agreement on ways to interpret diagnostic questions used in mental state examinations, such as 'Do you hear voices?', are of huge value.

WHEN CHALLENGING BEHAVIOUR CHALLENGES THE INTERPRETER

HIGHLY CHARGED MATERIAL

When verbal and non-verbal communication is highly charged, interpreters face many challenges. Interpreters sometimes find themselves unwittingly shielding the Deaf client by easing the emotional tenor of the discourse, for example when a patient is being admonished. Weigand (2000) feels the interpreter may inadvertently soften their delivery to either protect the patient's feelings or because of their own personal baggage. Napier and Cornes (2004) question the interpreter's impartiality in the face of emotional reaction to clients' material. They postulate that emotional loading may be greater if the interpreter is part of the Deaf community. For example, an interpreter who is a CODA (child of Deaf adults) may have witnessed their parents being oppressed because of their deafness and may therefore find it difficult to remain impartial if they are interpreting a situation where they feel the Deaf person present is also being oppressed.

In such situations a team comprising a hearing and Deaf interpreter, familiar with co-working, may usefully monitor each other's performance to guard against 'toning down' or overidentification with the patient.

Case Study Four

A hearing clinician rapidly presenting unpalatable information to a patient misunderstood the rather tetchy patient's response and made an unwelcome reply. The patient protested angrily. The interpreter tried to explain why he felt there had been a misunderstanding and asked for permission to check. The patient refused to repeat the conversation and his demeanour and delivery became threatening. Rather than provide a voiceover that echoed the patient's hostile manner, the interpreter chose to interpret the content accurately but lessen the tone, while informing the clinician that the patient, as a result of being completely misunderstood, was becoming aggressive. The interpreter had felt that had they mirrored the patient's mood and voiced a hostile tone, the clinician may have become defensive and the communication may have continued to break down. Using a calm voice to alert the clinician to the importance of addressing the misunderstanding resulted in the clinician being able to defuse the situation. The interpreter may have been torn between objectivity and role transgression in order to maintain calm in the session.

Some material is easier to interpret than others. When a patient is emotionally highly charged, they may be less able to tolerate lengthy clarifications or repetitions. If an interpreter is completing a lengthy voiceover to a hearing clinician, they may sign 'hold on' to the patient to allow themselves time to catch up. This sign in BSL involves a clenched fist directed at the patient. In these potentially explosive situations, this sign could at best be seen as rude or, at worst, threatening. Just as humility is required in hearing members of staff to decide whether they are capable of signing for themselves, so must the interpreter be aware of their own limitations. It is the authors' opinion that less experienced hearing interpreters leave it too long before admitting their difficulties, by which time the situation has escalated.

Whether an interpreter is working alone or in a relay team, it is imperative that time is taken for the clinician to brief them and for potential emotional and psychological reactions to be discussed. Napier and Cornes (2004) propose that therapy can only be enhanced by interpreters and therapists adopting flexible roles and working symbiotically.

THE INTERPRETER IN PHYSICAL DANGER

In escalating or threatening situations, the interpreter can feel vulnerable, since it is they who are actually delivering the message. However, in the authors' experience, this personal vulnerability is decreased by regularly indicating that it is someone else who is the source of the message.

In formal interpreting situations, the interpreter should only be present with the patient when the clinician is present. However, even with the best intentions, the clinician may need to leave the room, which leaves the interpreter alone with a potentially challenging patient. It should be made clear to mental health professionals that British and American interpreter codes of practice advise that interpreters should not remain alone with a patient (Registry of Interpreters for the Deaf, 2000; ASLI, 2005). The clinician should also be prepared to brief the interpreter beforehand regarding the goals of the interaction and inform them if the patient has a history of challenging behaviour. If potential for risk exists, the interpreter should ensure their exit path is free.

Interpreters may not routinely be given alarms, nor may they routinely do the same personal-safety training as staff. If an interpreter suffers injury while working for a hospital, they may have to claim against the hospital for compensation. Interpreters are generally covered by professional indemnity insurance, but this cover only applies in the case of professional error. Issues regarding health and safety need to be discussed with hospital authorities.

Professional supervision, debriefing or peer-support schemes need to be available to support interpreters who work in this field (ASLI, 2005).

THE ROLE OF INTERPRETERS DURING RESTRAINT

Occasionally, restraint procedures occur in mental health settings. This involves the patient being physically handled, usually against their will, for the safety of either themselves or others. Consideration must be given to the fundamental needs of the individual under restraint, and human rights legislation must still be adhered to during restraint (HMSO, 1998; National Institute for Clinical Excellence, 2005). Within this, legislation is the right of Deaf people to be free to communicate or to have access to some form of communication.

Hearing interpreters are rarely called for during restraint, but in the absence of Deaf staff or a Deaf interpreter they may want to volunteer to facilitate fair communication. In the heat of the moment, hearing staff may not think to use an interpreter until the crisis is over.

While in the UK neither the interpreters' codes formulated by the Council for the Advancement of Communication with Deaf people (CACDP) nor the Association of Sign Language Interpreters give direct guidance here, the authors contend that an interpreter in these circumstances should inform staff that they are available to interpret. During a restraint, the interpreter should be prepared to be flexible about where they operate. If the patient is being restrained on the floor, the interpreter may also need to be on the floor lying on their side to be visible to the patient. The interpreter may need to encourage the patient to look at them so they can communicate effectively.

The use of any form of restraint applied to the hands will restrict communication, whereas holding just the arms allows some hand move-ment. If the hands are held, the interpreter may need to explain to clinicians that the patient is being prevented from communicating. It is not always possible to voice-over the patient's speech, which may be, or may have become, unintelligible. Interpreter codes state that inter-preters should not assist in physical restraint (Registry of Interpreters for the Deaf, 2000; ASLI, 2005). Interpreters may feel powerless if they see a restraint that they think is too rough, but they do have the rights and the responsibility, as does any citizen, to approach the hospital complaints department or the police if they think a patient has been treated unlawfully.

THE PROBLEM OF BLURRED BOUNDARIES: INTERPRETER OR SNEAK?

Pollard (1997) advises that, if the interpreter's special language or cultural knowledge leads them to suspect that a situation is becoming unstable or dangerous and the clinician seems to be unaware of this, it is important to pass this on. In the authors' opinion, this is not clear-cut. For the Deaf employee (for example a nursing assistant or psychologist) their responsibility to respond to this is clear. For the interpreter, whether freelance or employee, it is not so clear.

Interpreters are usually expected to interpret in pre-arranged settings such as clinical interviews and are not required to spontaneously volunteer information that they have 'overheard' (a fact that they have seen which was not directly communicated to them). However, their role as facilitator of social communication within, for example, a mental health day centre puts them in a position to 'overhear' material that could be vital to staff and patient safety.

Certainly, Deaf interpreters and some highly skilled interpreters will be able to monitor exchanges between patients and recognise sign codes that give clues about dynamics, relationships, hierarchies, bullying and other behaviours. This level of comprehension enables true monitoring and allows staff to pick up early signs of frustration and put measures in place to prevent escalation. However, the interpreter's position is tricky. Under the Health and Safety at Work Act (HMSO, 1974), the interpreter has to decide whether the information they overhear is related to risk or not: a decision they may not be qualified or informed enough to make. Interpreters in the UK working on hospital premises are bound by this Act to have a duty of care to all stakeholders with whom they have contact which include staff and visitors as well as patients. If an interpreter withholds information about a patient's intended behaviour and that behaviour poses a risk to the patient or others, the interpreter is in breach of this duty. Regular and ongoing formal dialogue between interpreters and the mental health service team is necessary to address these kinds of dilemmas.

Within this chapter, we have suggested ways in which the interpreter can assist in day-to-day communication between hearing staff and Deaf patients. However, these interventions require the interpreter to be based within the patients' space when they are not involved in a specific interpreting task. The interpreter and mental health team need to jointly decide whether the benefit of the ever-present interpreter outweighs the difficulties arising from the interpreter having to make unilateral judgements as to the degree of risk 'overheard' material represents.

CONCLUSION

Several issues have been highlighted that show how the quality of the communication environment within a Deaf mental health service affects the occurrence of challenging behaviour. Sign language training must be a priority, and staff should be encouraged to create a non-threatening communication environment where everyone feels comfortable to practise their communication skills and to maximise the involvement of the Deaf client. By improving the communication environment and the acceptance of Deaf culture, Deaf staff and interpreters have a role in reducing and managing challenging behaviour. The adaptive linguistic skills of Deaf staff are of such value in these situations that financial and career package rewards are needed to improve their recruitment and retention.

Making full use of the Deaf relay interpreter requires a certain amount of humility on the part of the hearing clinician or hearing interpreter. However, in the authors' experience, the opportunity to de-escalate or prevent challenging behaviour is often related to how comfortable hearing staff are to use a relay interpreter.

Interpreting in situations where there is challenging behaviour has many challenges for the hearing interpreter and Deaf relay interpreter. Pertinent issues include the interpreter's own safety, the ability to translate accurately in a highly charged arena and the interpreter's role, via communication access, in protecting the human rights of the patient. Full briefing of interpreters is essential and structured team discussions regarding dilemmas and practice are invaluable. The development of interpreter training in mental health and specifically in challenging behaviour is essential.

REFERENCES

ASLI (2005) *Draft Code of Practice for Sign Language Interpreters Working in Mental Health (Draft 9)*, London, Association of Sign Language Interpreters of England, Wales and Northern Ireland, http://www.asli.org.uk/documents/codeofpractiseforinterpretersinmentalhealth.pdf, accessed 14 March 2006.

Conrad R (1979) *The Deaf School Child*, London, Harper and Row.

Department of Health (2000) *The NHS Plan: A Plan for Investment; A Plan for Reform*, London' TSO.

Du Feu M, Fergusson K (2003) Sensory impairment and mental health. *Advances in Psychiatric Treatment* 9(2): 95–103.

Gregory RJ, Canning SS, Lee TW, Wise JC (2004) Cognitive bibliotherapy for depression: a meta-analysis. *Professional Psychology: Research and Practice* 35(3): 275–80.

Hamerdinger S, Karlin B (2003) Therapy using interpreters: question on the use of interpreters in therapeutic settings for monolingual therapists. *Journal of the American Deafness and Rehabilitation Association* 36(3): 12–30.

HMSO (1974) Health and Safety at Work Act 1974, available from http://www.opsi.gov.uk/si/si2001/20012127.htm., accessed 23 February 2006.

HMSO (1998) *The Human Rights Act 1998*, London, TSO.

Kitson N, Austen S (2004) Mental health services for deaf people. In Austen S and Crocker S (eds), *Deafness In Mind: Working Psychologically with Deaf People Across the Lifespan*, London, Whurr, pp. 147–60.

Kitson N, Klein H (2000) Mental health workers: deaf-hearing partnerships. In Hindley P and Kitson N (eds), *Mental Health and Deafness*, London, Whurr, pp. 285–96.

Marcos LR (1979) Effects of interpreters on evaluation of psychopathology in non-English-speaking patients. *American Journal of Psychiatry* 136(2): 171–4.

Napier J, Cornes A (2004) The dynamic roles of interpreters and therapists. In Austen S and Crocker S (eds), *Deafness In Mind: Working Psychologically with Deaf People Across the Lifespan*, London, Whurr, pp. 161–79.

National Institute for Clinical Excellence (2005) *Short-term Management of Violent/Disturbed Behaviour in In-Patient Psychiatric Settings and Emergency Departments*, London, TSO.

Pollard RQ (1997) *Mental Health Interpreting: A Mentored Curriculum*, Rochester NY, University of Rochester.

Registry of Interpreters for the Deaf (2000) *Interpreting in Mental Health Settings*, Rochester, VA, RID.

Ridgeway SM (1997) Deaf people and psychology: some preliminary findings. *Deaf Worlds* 13(1): 9–17.

Steinberg MD, Sullivan VJ, Loew RC (1998) Cultural and linguistic barriers to mental health service access: the deaf consumer's perspective. *American Journal of Psychiatry* 155(7): 982–4.

Taylor L (2002) Defining the shadow: recognising the imprint of the interpreter in the mental health setting. In Gutman V (ed), *Ethics in Mental Health and Deafness*, Washington, Gallaudet University Press, pp. 123–48.

Watson D, Williams V, Wickham C, Kyle J, Dury A (2005) *Final Report on the Sequal Project on Employment and Disabled People*, Guildford, The Sequal DP.

Weigand C (2000) Role of the interpreter in the healing of a nation: an emotional view. In Roberts RP, Carr SE, Abraham D, Dufour A (eds), *The Critical Link 2. Interpreters in the Community*, Amsterdam, John Benjamins, pp. 207–18.

14

Social-skills Improvement as a Means of Managing Challenging Behavior

MARLENE EERNISSE AND LEIGH POOLE WARREN

INTRODUCTION

Historically, service-oriented professions have not participated in transdisciplinary approaches to treatment. A psychologist and speech/language pathologist (SLP) team has been established to more effectively address behavioral deficits that may be a manifestation of a language delay. Using role-play, peer collaboration and reciprocal teaching, chronic maladaptive behaviors are discussed and analyzed for evidence of good decision-making and critical thinking. In addition, language is taught to improve social interactions and to decrease the frustrations resulting from communication breakdowns.

THE LINKS BETWEEN LANGUAGE AND CHALLENGING BEHAVIOR

LANGUAGE, VERBAL AND VOCABULARY SKILLS

The inherent language difficulties of individuals with hearing loss make addressing pragmatic deficits increasingly problematic. Deaf children

Deafness and Challenging Behaviour: The 360° Perspective. Edited by S. Austen and D. Jeffery
© 2007 John Wiley & Sons Ltd

exposed to conversational rules of English and American Sign Language (ASL) simultaneously may not be able to discern the appropriate context in which to use discretion. One overwhelming deficit is the individual's lack of vocabulary to express their feelings and frustrations. This deficit can, anecdotally, be blamed for many of the behavioral outbursts observed.

The major components of a language system include syntax, the rules for developing sentences; semantics, the meaning of words; and pragmatics, the rules for conversational use. The components represent the form, content and use of language. A child with a hearing impairment receives a weakened speech signal, which adversely affects his or her ability to acquire information regarding the form, content and use of language. The subsequent result is a language delay (Seyfried and Kricos, 1996).

The semantic skills of a child with a hearing impairment may vary greatly; however, the majority of children with hearing loss exhibit vocabulary skills that are lower than those of their same-aged hearing peers. Many of the programs that address the language needs of children with hearing loss are centered on vocabulary development and syntax rather than targeting functional communication skills (Seyfried and Kricos, 1996). To fill this gap, activities are used to help develop social competence. Antia and Kreimeyer (1992) define social competence as the ability to communicate by using a common symbol system and by understanding the guidelines for communication in diverse social situations.

According to Cartwright *et al.* (1989), carrying on conversations is a characteristic that is unique to human beings. Children that exhibit delayed speech and language skills may experience a lifetime of difficulty communicating in an acceptable manner. Training focused on pragmatic skills may be instrumental in aiding specific skill development.

Pragmatics of a given language system can be defined as the strategies and knowledge for appropriate eye contact, initiation and termination of conversations, repair of communication breakdowns, topic shifts and turn-taking. By targeting specific pragmatic aspects of English, the goal is to assist individuals so that they improve social skills as well as their overall world knowledge. Research indicates that many children with hearing loss experience difficulty with turn-taking, topic initiation and maintenance; however, there appears to be a steady increase in the aforementioned skills as the child becomes more fluent in ASL (Seyfried and Kricos, 1996).

SOCIAL SKILLS

Brinton and Fujiki (1993) suggest that approximately 10% of children may not have typically developing social skills. Most likely, this approximation would increase in the population of children with disabilities. Typically developing children mature through phases of learning language.

- They will begin by using language to make their wants and needs known.
- The second phase is using language to recognize specific emotions in themselves and in others.
- Then, the child will use language to learn how to control the emotions, and use this knowledge in social settings.

For children with limited access to language, vocabulary of emotions or situations requiring specific social skills, this lack of experience can lead to maladaptive behaviors. Giddan *et al.* (1995) suggest there is high probability that children with language deficiencies will also have disorders relating to social behavior. These behaviors may be manifested in numerous ways. Children might exhibit depression and be withdrawn, or be extremely active, aggressive and/or volatile. In the past, criteria have been established to identify children with language disorders. However, special services that have been provided to treat language disorders tend to exclude co-morbid disorders, such as retardation, sensory impairment and emotional disorders (Brinton and Fujiki, 1993).

In the hearing world, social skills as common as acknowledging a person in a hallway are taken for granted. Most children assimilate social behaviors easily because they are exposed to them from infancy. As early as possible, adults expect children to exchange social hellos and goodbyes by waving long before speech occurs. Deaf children do not receive this stimulation in the same degrees as hearing children and therefore might not be aware of the behaviors expected of them while still being held to those standards. Antia and Kreimeyer (1992) used an intervention program to practice specific social skills with hearing-impaired children aged three to four. The focus was on the following skills: greeting peers, sharing materials, assisting, complimenting and praising, cooperative play and inviting. Results indicated the children exhibited an overall increase in positive interactions among their peer groups.

CULTURAL BRIDGE

Because society comprises a variety of cultures, it is important to instil a sense of tolerance, sensitivity and acceptance toward cultural practices that differ from those personally experienced. Individuals perceiving themselves as culturally deaf need a working knowledge of the differences in hearing culture as they transition from a deaf environment to a hearing environment. The program facilitators want to expand the world knowledge of the participants to ease this integration. This process begins by exposing the cultural norms for hearing and deaf individuals. Often there is a lack of experience and knowledge regarding these differences. Without the 'cultural bridge', the likelihood of challenging behavior is heightened.

It should be noted that hearing and deaf cultures are not the only barriers present. Once a working knowledge of racial, ethnic and cultural differences is obtained, scenarios can be role-played to examine different outcomes.

DECISION-MAKING AND CRITICAL THINKING

When working with children with challenging behavior and language difficulties, the authors give a great amount of focus to critical thinking and decision-making. This is done through discussions which are designed to help an individual start with an action, think through all of the options available to him or her and the options available to any other individuals involved and to follow the actions chosen out to their natural conclusion. In this way, the decision-making process can be looked at carefully and critically in a low-stress environment and decisions that have undesirable results can be examined. The goal is to create a bridge between the low-stress sessions and the solutions discovered there and high-stress situations where critical thinking and good decision-making are crucial. If the participant is able to think through his or her actions before engaging in some variety of maladaptive behavior, the outcome of the crisis situation may be more desirable.

Case Study: Joe

Joe is a student who has received behavioral services since he was a small child for problems ranging from aggression and destruction of property to stealing and emotional outbursts. While there have been some areas of vast improvement, Joe continues to exhibit problematic behavior, primarily due to below-average intelligence and poor judgment. He is an easy scapegoat for other students and finds himself in undesirable situations due to his need for peer acceptance. One of the most serious incidents that involved Joe was setting a trash can on fire in a classroom during class. Other students, who were angry with the teacher, persuaded Joe to set the fire so they could not be blamed. The other students involved were perceived by Joe as popular. They were all upperclassmen, and Joe was eager to earn their acceptance. The other students convinced Joe that his participation made him part of the group. This perception of camaraderie motivated Joe to act.

After this particularly serious incident, Joe was referred to the school psychologist for counseling. Since individuals are never referred to the school psychologist for positive reasons, Joe was immediately nervous and defensive. No amount of reassurance would calm Joe or convince him that he was not in new trouble. Most sessions terminated with him in distress, perceiving he had been accused of more misdeeds. Finally, after multiple attempts, counseling was discontinued for the last few weeks of the school year. A new strategy was needed when the new school year began because the problems remained.

Joe had worked with the same SLP for four years. They had a solid rapport and he found her therapy room to be a non-threatening environment. Gradually, over the course of several sessions, the psychologist integrated into their normal work and routine. Then, using worksheets similar to those used previously, some speech/language sessions shifted focus to increasing his behavior vocabulary in an attempt to give him sufficient skills to express his feelings. In addition, the psychologist and SLP engaged in role-play scenarios with Joe as observer and analyst. Since he was not portrayed as an offender, he was able to remain focused on the situation, openly identify feelings that might be instrumental in the decision-making process and discuss the different behavior choices that were available. This approach to co-treatment enabled Joe to participate in psychological sessions without experiencing feelings of anxiety. Success was evident in that his behavioral problems the following school year were relatively minor and infrequent.

JOINT WORKING

Traditionally, individuals in need of special services such as speech and language therapy, occupational therapy, physical therapy, psychological services, social work services and tutoring have received support to address the needs that are discipline specific. Recent research, such as the study on collaborative partnerships completed by Prelock *et al.* (1995), indicates that using a transdisciplinary approach to treatment yields more effective outcomes than individual professionals providing services solely within their discipline. A team approach uses the skills and knowledge of the professions involved but does not breach the parameters that define their scope of practice.

Efforts are being made to improve the effectiveness of support services in the areas of behavior modification and speech/language therapy. To address this issue, a team comprising the authors, a psychologist and an SLP, used co-treatment group sessions to target specific pragmatic aspects of English in which the students exhibited a delay.

JOINT PSYCHOLOGY AND SPEECH/THERAPY PROGRAM

CLIENT GROUP

With personal knowledge of the students, their personalities and the issues that need to be addressed, the psychologist and SLP team reviewed the student roster and decided which students to include in the initial groups. Referrals from teachers were taken into consideration. Formation of groups focused on social-skill needs, functioning level, language abilities, maturity level and/or grade level. Groups were also formed based on common chronic maladaptive behaviors. Accommodations were made for teachers requesting that specific students or entire classes be included as a group. As a means of behavior support, continuing efforts were made to include any individual having sporadic behavioral issues. Owing to differences in residual hearing, auditory perceptual skills and varying abilities to speech read, all sessions were conducted in ASL.

PROGRAM STRUCTURE

The groups were specifically designed to address emotion-based language, general conversational skills and independent/critical thinking.

Co-treatment sessions explored the vast array of emotions and events that may elicit the emergence of each emotion and the appropriate ways to express that emotion. Within the group program, the following features/techniques, taken from the repertoire of Schunk (2004), were practiced:

- transfer
- self-regulation
- reciprocal teaching
- peer collaboration.

Transfer

'Transfer' refers to new knowledge and skills that are being applied in different situations than those in which they were obtained. Therefore, role-play is used to emulate a variety of stressful situations.

Self-regulation

'Self-regulation' is the term given to the process on which individuals purposefully direct their thoughts, behaviors and choices toward the achievement of personally set goals. In addition, these sessions are intended to help equip the individuals with the appropriate language to aid them in communicating their wants, needs, feelings and concerns with accuracy and clarity.

Reciprocal Teaching

The evolution of this program has transitioned from individual sessions in favor of group sessions using Vygotsky's (1978) ideas of reciprocal teaching and peer collaboration. 'Reciprocal teaching' involves a dialogue between a teacher and a student or a group of students. The teacher models the desired behavior and then each student acts as the teacher and reinstructs the group on that behavior.

Peer Collaboration

'Peer collaboration' fosters a positive group dynamic. Research indicates that cooperative groups have the greatest effect when each student has a specific responsibility that must be accomplished for the success of the group as a whole. The current emphasis is on using peer groups for learning in fields such as mathematics, science and language arts; this gives credence to the importance of the social environment during learning.

THE CO-TREATMENT METHOD

> We spend a considerable amount of time telling students with disabilities, who display inappropriate behavior, what to do, and what not to do. We sometimes forgot to tell them how to achieve what we ask of them, or we take for granted a communication problem. Students may not understand what it is you are asking. Other times they may not see the need for changing their behavior and, still other times, the students are just not capable of performing what we tell them to do. We need to tell them how to deal with the feelings they are experiencing. (Zimmerman, 2001, p. 225)

Co-treatment sessions fill this need by going into specific instances that might elicit negative behaviour or poor decision-making, and all options are weighed and discussed. In therapy sessions, conversations are practiced. One student initiates a topic and, under the therapist's guidance, turn-taking occurs and the topic is maintained. Also, groups may discuss appropriate eye contact, social behaviors and the situations in which these are used.

Situations are set up, explained and enacted. Each possibility is dramatized, and a conversation follows about which choices bring the most desirable results and which ones bring less desirable results. Most sessions begin by identifying language common to the session's theme. For example, if the theme is independent thinking, common words or phrases are written, explained and discussed in the hopes that the individual will store this information and use it as needed.

In ASL, some words have multiple signs depending on meaning. One example of this is 'make'. There are multiple signs for the word 'make': make lunch, make money and make a person do something, and so on. ASL skills are strengthened by the determination of meaning and the explanation of why a particular sign is used. This also strengthens reading, comprehension and communication skills.

Zimmerman encapsulates the aims of a group such as this.

> By giving these individuals strategies and providing a tool belt, or coping strategies, we assist them in making positive choices. It would be foolish to assume that during every situation an individual will pick a strategy from his or her tool belt. However, if we don't give them a tool belt, they will never have the option of choosing. (Zimmerman, 2001, p. 229)

THERAPY SESSION EXAMPLES

Perhaps this method can best be explained by real examples of therapy sessions. The authors have translated these conversations, which took place in ASL, into more standard English so that the meanings would be clear.

While taking the annual statewide test, Marcus, a sixth grader, was being disruptive. Marcus had tested significantly below grade level in all academic areas and was obviously frustrated by his inability to complete test items. The test administrator made numerous attempts to get Marcus to cooperate, but to no avail. The test proctor tried to convince him to go to the principal's office. Marcus perceived this as punishment and his behavior worsened to the point of verbal and physical aggression directed at the school principal. The event culminated in suspension.

Upon Marcus' return to school, he was in a group session that discussed the incident. The whole situation was analyzed step by step and the choices available at each critical juncture were discussed. For example, when Marcus realized that he did not understand the test questions, his options were to ask for ASL interpretation, sit quietly until the next test section began, bother other students or run out of the room. Marcus indicated that he understood there were many options open to him. Discussion of each option included consideration of each possible outcome. Marcus and the group members were able to correctly predict and identify which options and outcomes were positive and negative. The group was asked which emotions were present and how they related to the sequence of events. The group participated by giving examples of words Marcus could have used to better communicate with the test administrator regarding his frustration.

In review, the therapists write down certain words and phrases that have previously been explained so the group members will have the opportunity to use specific ASL signs that indicate comprehension of a concept. To achieve session continuity, a review of vocabulary and concepts previously discussed occur at the onset of each session.

CONCLUSION

Evidence suggests that children with language delays may exhibit increased problematic behaviors and more poorly developed social skills than their typically developing peers. The problematic behaviors can be addressed by correctly identifying the underlying language deficits. By integrating the skills of professionals in psychology and SLP, the delayed components of language may be more readily identified and effectively addressed. The goal is to increase the individual's ability to identify options that may lead to positive outcomes and more successful social interactions.

REFERENCES

Antia S, Kreimeyer K (1992) Social competence intervention for young children with hearing impairments. In Odom S, McConnell S, McEvoy M (eds), *Social Competence in Young Children with Disabilities: Issues and Strategies for Intervention*, Baltimore, Paul H Brookes, pp. 135–64.

Brinton B, Fujiki M (1993) Clinical forum: language and social skills in the school-age population language, social skills, and socioemotional behavior. *Language, Speech and Hearing Services in Schools* 24(4): 194–8.

Cartwright G, Cartwright C, Ward M (1989) *Educating Special Learners* (3rd edn.), Belmont, CA, Wadsworth.

Giddan J, Bade K, Rickenberg D, Ryley A (1995) Teaching the language of feelings to students with severe emotional and behavioral handicaps. *Language, Speech and Hearing Services in Schools* 26(1): 3–10.

Prelock P, Miller B, Reed N (1995) Collaborative partnerships in language in the classroom program. *Language, Speech and Hearing Services in Schools* 26(3): 286–92.

Schunk D (2004) *Learning Theories: An Educational Perspective* (4th edn.), Englewood Cliffs, NJ, Prentice Hall.

Seyfried D, Kricos P (1996) Language and speech of the deaf and hard-of-hearing. In Schow R, Nerbonne M (eds), *Introduction to Audiologic Rehabilitation* (3rd edn.), Boston, Allyn and Bacon, pp. 168–228.

Vygotsky LS (1978) *Mind in Society: The Development of Higher Psychological Processes*, Cambridge, MA, Harvard University Press.

Zimmerman B (2001) *Why Can't They Just Behave? A Guide to Managing Student Behavior Disorders*, Harsham, PA, LRP Publications.

15

Approach with Care: Improving the Effectiveness of the Care Programme Approach with Deaf Service Users in the UK

DAVE JEFFERY

INTRODUCTION

The Care Programme Approach (CPA), when underpinned by appropriate risk assessment, risk management and a recovery-based ethos, will help support service users, their carers and local generic mental health professionals (MHP) to effectively manage challenging behaviour (CB). However, CPA has been inconsistently applied within the UK (Simpson *et al.*, 2003). The Department of Heath (DH) has conceded that logistics play a major factor in the effectiveness of the CPA when specialist deaf mental health services attempt to work across large geographic areas (DH, 2005).

The ramifications of poor implementation of CPA can be illustrated by tragedies and their subsequent inquiries spanning twenty years (Department of Health and Social Security, 1988; Ritchie, 1994; Mishcon *et al.*, 2000). To use CPA effectively, regional specialist mental health services for deaf people need to work innovatively.

Deafness and Challenging Behaviour: The 360° Perspective. Edited by S. Austen and D. Jeffery
© 2007 John Wiley & Sons Ltd

This chapter will introduce a brief history of CPA, the factors that underpin its design and its short falls. The author recommends a single point of entry referral process, involving trained Gateway Workers, to improve the interface between specialist deaf mental health services and local (generic) mental health services. A recovery-based approach is suggested to complement the CPA process in the management of CB in both hearing and deaf people.

ESTABLISHING THE NEED FOR CPA: AN HISTORICAL PERSPECTIVE

Warner suggests that CPA can be considered as:

> a type of case management albeit one not based on a specific case management model (Warner, 2005, p. 2)

The ethos of CPA was derived from such case management systems initiated in North America during the 1970s. Case management was a series of frameworks and models that allowed for the consistent and effective delivery of healthcare services (Mueser *et al.*, 1998).

The need for CPA in the UK originated from an overwhelming recognition for coordinated community mental health services (Audit Commission, 1986). In the mid- to late eighties, haphazard and often inconsistent community arrangements prompted an acknowledgement that service users with severe mental illnesses (SMI) should expect better care post discharge (Wallace, 1986). The subsequent inquiry into the death of a social worker at the hands of a female service user with SMI reported that non-concordance with mental health services had been a contributory factor, concluding that a register of vulnerable persons was needed (Department of Health and Social Security, 1988). The report suggested a nominated keyworker allocated to each person upon such a register.

In response to this, the Griffiths Report (1988) suggested more structured responsibilities for the keyworker (or in this instance: case worker) role. Care packages were to be specific to the fundamental needs of the individual service user, arrived at following careful assessment, then organising and coordinating the agencies involved in the care package as a result of the formulated care plan.

The Department of Health and Social Security (DHSS) White Paper *Caring for People* (DHSS, 1989) may have been heavily informed by the Griffiths Report but the publication's emphasis upon mental health was swamped by the anticipation of further legislation. The National Health Service and Community Care Act (DH, 1990a) aimed to enforce radical reform within in-patient and community mental health services.

As local social service authorities pressed on with case management systems, a DH circular was issued cautioning psychiatrists not to discharge their service users without an agreed plan of care and the involvement of the local authority (DH, 1990b).

By 1990, it was the expectation that all service users referred to mental health services should be considered eligible for CPA (DH, 1990c). Throughout the nineties, however, CPA was not applied with the consistency required to make it effective (Audit Commission, 1994). Warner (2005) notes that despite the CPA being considered the mechanism by which mental health services could be delivered in a standardised fashion this level of uniformity did not extend to the fabric of implementation. As such, many health authorities held their own interpretation of how to integrate the system within their locality.

The DH publication *Building Bridges* (DH, 1995) offered further guidance on interagency working but failed to enforce a unified method on an operational level, save for the suggestion that the approach could be tiered, with only individuals with complex issues requiring full multidisciplinary CPA.

Revised in 1999, the CPA incorporated care management, with the intention to firm up the health and social care elements of the process (DH, 1999a). Individuals of a working age with mental health needs would now receive an assessment, be given a formulated care plan by a designated care coordinator (replacing the keyworker role) and expect such a plan to be reviewed regularly. This strategy would be completed by both health and social care staff. These arrangements included in-patient services. The CPA tiers were also standardised. Nationally, there were to be only two categories of CPA: standard and enhanced. Figure 15.1 illustrates the criteria of each tier.

NATIONAL SUPPORTIVE GUIDANCE

The DH concedes that the revision of CPA was prompted by factors pertaining to its original design and the climate of change forged by the modernisation agenda (DH, 1997, 1998, 1999b).

The *National Service Framework for Mental Health* (DH, 1999b) makes implicit reference to the CPA. Standard four demands that the

Standard CPA Elements	Enhanced CPA Elements
• single agency involvement	• multiple care needs requiring multi-agency involvement/coordination
• low level of involvement from one or more agency	• require frequent and intensive intervention
• self-management of mental health issues	
• low risk of danger to self or others	• high risk of harming self or others
• concordant with input from services	• non-concordant with service input

Figure 15.1 Criteria for Standard and Enhanced CPA (Adapted from Warner, 2005)

service user can expect a copy of their written care plan that includes a list of contact details of the professionals involved in their care and an action plan as to what professionals and carers should do in the event of a crisis. This is completed and regularly updated by the care coordinator. The importance of the CPA is reiterated in *Code of Practice: Mental Health Act (1983)* (DH and Welsh Office, 1999) when service users are discharged from a stay in hospital under the Act.

PROBLEMS WITH THE IMPLEMENTATION OF CPA (GENERIC PERSPECTIVE)

As there have been ongoing issues with the implementation of CPA from its inception, it is not surprising that even with major reforms deficits still remain. It has been identified that the efficiency of both CPA and risk management relies upon the systematic flux of information communicated between all agencies (DH, 1999a).

Simpson *et al.* (2003) note problems with interagency discourse as being a contributory factor in the failings of the successful integration and implementation of CPA. According to Barre and Evans (2005), multi-agency team working is seen by many as a major obstacle to the effective delivery of care. Some argue that the pooling of differing professional perspectives and experiences can only add to the collaborative process that is CPA (Miller *et al.*, 2001). Yet it has been suggested that professional culture and organisational constraints are primary catalysts for impaired practice (Peck and Norman, 1999).

Far from creating the unified cohesive system it sought, CPA has been criticised as becoming divisive. Simpson *et al.* (2003) argue that a failure to reinforce the clinical merits of CPA negated its value amongst MHPs, who perceived the tool as causing potential friction within their relationships with service users. At an intrinsic level, the therapeutic alliance has potential to become compromised as MHPs struggle to balance the dual role of coordinator and practitioner (May, 1996; Rush, 2004).

Anthony and Crawford (2000) believe that the basic disparity in the statutory obligations of the MHP and the consumerist ideologies that pervade the modernisation agenda may reinforce this issue. Few studies have examined this complex and potentially contradictory relationship, despite the importance of such factors in undermining fundamental practice.

McDermott (1998) observes that the many service users do not feel that they are integral to the design of their care package. In principle at least, service user involvement in service planning and care delivery has been at the heart of healthcare reform for over fifteen years, but it has been noted that true collaboration has fallen foul to incongruity in government macro- and micro-policy (Rush, 2004). As a consequence, service user involvement may have been unwittingly impeded by the risk-management and statutory elements of CPA. This will be discussed further with reference to the **recovery paradigm** (p. 245).

RISK ASSESSMENT AS A CORE PRINCIPLE OF CPA

It is impossible to discuss CPA without an acknowledgement of its role in the protection of the public. As a systematic tool for delivering mental health services, CPA is commonly absent or poorly implemented when tragedy occurs (Shepherd, 1996; DHSS, 1988).

CPA operates within clear clinical risk-management and clinical risk-assessment philosophies. The DH makes it clear that:

> Risk assessment is an essential and ongoing part of the CPA process. (DH, 1999a, p. 7)

CPA in isolation is not a risk-assessment tool. It is merely a framework that captures the core elements of risk in order to formulate a clinical risk strategy for the individual service user. It should be noted that the eradication of risk in delivering mental health services, while admirable, is recognised as being an unrealistic expectation (DH, 1999a). The primary focus of risk assessment and subsequent risk management is the reduction and minimisation of potential risks. Risk assessment has been identified by the Health and Safety Executive (HSE) as:

> a careful examination of what, in your work, could cause harm to people, so that you can weigh up whether you have taken enough precautions or should do more to prevent harm (HSE, 2003, p. 2)

An important influence upon the effectiveness of any risk-management strategy is a good working knowledge of the process. An established process for risk assessment is given below. The importance of risk assessment is that it should be ongoing, a factor that was highlighted in the reform of CPA in the late nineties (DH, 1999a). The key areas of the risk-assessment process are (HSE, 2003):

1. Identify the hazard
2. Identify who may be affected by the hazard
3. Evaluate the risks
4. Record your findings
5. Review and revise

A shortfall has been identified in the calibre of education in risk management for MHPs acting as care coordinators and expected to work within the CPA (May, 1996). This has an implication for awareness in other areas of risk management considering that public, and to some degree professional, perceptions of 'risk' involve danger. But practitioners must still acknowledge that other factors will also play a role in shaping an individual's behaviour, for example financial and social needs.

CPA suggests that risk reduction in this context relates to specific actions and arrangements that comprise a crisis-management and a relapse (warning signs) plan. This is used to identify and incorporate factors that are poignant in the prevention, prediction and management of individual risk behaviours.

DEAF MENTAL HEALTH SERVICES

The National Deaf Mental Health Service (NDMHS) in Birmingham functions on a regional level. It is designed to offer services to support primary care (GPs etc.) and community mental health trusts (CMHTs) to deliver services to the local deaf population. The benefit of such a service to the deaf service user is clear: access to mental health services that reflect their unique linguistic and cultural needs. Local services benefit from a resource that will assist in the accurate mental health assessment of a deaf person and support local MHPs to manage their care accordingly.

Local CMHTs often assume that the NDMHS provides all aspects of mental health service. There have been examples within the NDMHS of local teams discharging deaf service users once they have been offered an appointment with, or admitted to, an in-patient bed in the NDMHS. In these instances, the initial mental health assessment has been construed as the secondary, as opposed to tertiary, care process. In these situations, a process of pressured negotiation has ensued to recommence local services so that joint work can take place or that the deaf person can be discharged safely.

CPA IN DEAF MENTAL HEALTH SERVICES

In 1998, Daniel Joseph, a deaf service user under the care of the National Deaf Service (NDS), London, killed his neighbour Carla Thompson and seriously injured Agnes Erume (Mishcon *et al.*, 2000). A key finding of this inquiry was that Daniel Joseph had no CPA documentation, and risk needs were not evaluated with adequate frequency.

The recommendations of Mishcon *et al.* (2000) indicate the need for a fundamental revision of collaborative practices not only within the deaf mental health services but also of how these services work with local and not-so-local agencies.

Recommendation 7 of the Daniel Joseph inquiry suggests that all deaf services make clear to the referring agency their responsibilities and purpose based upon:

agreed protocols but ultimately will depend on individual care plans (Mishcon *et al.*, 2000, p. 127)

The onus for change is placed upon the existing specialist deaf mental health services in the UK. The expectation is that these deaf services will support both the deaf service user and the local team involved with their care (DH, 2004). While the resource implications are acknowledged, the overall ethos is that of joint working irrespective of logistics (DH, 2005).

PROBLEMS WITH THE IMPLEMENTATION OF CPA (DEAF PERSPECTIVE)

The mere replication of existing frameworks that have not been adapted for use with the Deaf community presents service users and MHPs with several issues. It is reasonable to suggest that any care package needs to be designed in conjunction with the target client group. To work collaboratively requires a level of understanding of the CPA process and the documentation associated with it, as well as some knowledge of the client group. Many generic approaches have been made in the absence of Deaf-specific frameworks with varying degrees of success (Pollard, 2002). Existing tools can therefore lack cultural cogency, not recognising the intricacies of working with deaf people with SMI, and the practitioner's acceptance of their own deficits within this area (Peoples, 2002).

The principal concerns of CPA and deaf services centre on communication and logistics. This is due to the fundamental design of CPA being based upon immediate locality and how this impacts upon the established problems with mental health services for local Deaf communities (DH, 2004).

COMMUNICATION AND KNOWLEDGE OF DEAF CULTURE

Effective communication between local generic and national specialist teams is crucial to the success of CPA for deaf people. However, communication is also the keystone in the effective management of challenging behaviour (Emerson, 2001). The everyday frustrations experienced by a deaf person may be enough to trigger challenging behaviours. When coupled with factors related to inappropriate or inaccessible assessment and treatment, there may be a probability of an increase in existing maladaptive behaviours.

Often the local CMHT feels that it cannot meet the needs of deaf people because of the communication issues. However, this is a staggering failure of obligation to a minority group. This discrimination could be easily addressed by gaining Deaf awareness (training that is reasonably easy to access) or the acquisition of necessary communication skills.

LOGISTICS

A rudimentary method of examining the influence of logistics on CPA with deaf service users is to consider the core elements of the CPA framework, which are:

- assessment process
- care and crisis planning
- coordinating the care package
- reviewing the care package.

Assessment Process

When a regional specialist team operates within another locality, the assessment process can become problematic. Accurate assessment and design of an appropriate care plan may be hampered by unfamiliarity: with the deaf person, their family, the local MHP and with the services available to the service user locally.

Issues of confidentiality may arise as a consequence of language barriers as the service user and local MHPs rely upon the family to help formulate and interpret the assessment process. This may be influenced by a deaf person who cannot read being asked via the family to divulge personal information. Valuable subjective data that will ultimately inform the assessment process may be subsequently lost. The service user may also feel inhibited when talking about family dynamics if their relatives are in the room with them.

A common assumption is that care planning for deaf people assessed by the NDMHS immediately becomes their sole responsibility. If so, the local CMHT effectively hands over statutory responsibilities for a member of its own community.

Care and Crisis Planning

There is a current expectation the NDMHS hold care coordination for deaf people irrespective of distance. This issue has not been readily clarified in recent DH guidance (DH, 2005), but expectations laid out in DH (1999b), for example 24-hour access in times of crisis make it plain that this is neither credible nor viable for an effective CPA process.

The allocation of appropriate care professionals is imperative if any crisis plan is to be truly effective. The care plan should incorporate a sound knowledge of local services available to the service user in a crisis event. DH (1999b) makes clear the need for service users to have ready access to mental health services near to their home. Both regional and local services need to ensure that access mechanisms during times of crisis are both available and consistent. Traditionally, it has often been problematic for NDMHS to gain access to highly specialised crisis services of the local mental health service, such as assertive outreach and home treatment teams, who tend to discriminate on the grounds of communication.

DH (1999a) conclude that any risk management plan should include:

- the person the service user is most receptive to during crisis
- how this person should be contacted during points of crisis
- the identification of pre-existing strategies that have proven effective in the management of previous behaviour.

If this concept is to work effectively, it can be argued that local teams will be required to build their relationships with deaf service users. This will be especially important prior to and during times of crisis.

Coordinating the Care Package

If the concept of professional boundaries can cause issue within local teams (Peck and Norman, 1999), there is a sound argument that working with more than one team across large geographical areas will have similar or worse problems. The limits of the CPA within the concept of interregional working are simple enough. The process was designed to integrate health and social care at a local level. Reform of the CPA is tacit acknowledgement by the DH that there is a lack of local mental health service involvement, and yet more than an awareness of the problem is needed to satisfactorily solve the problem (DH, 2004, 2005).

The need for a care coordinator to be based within the service user's locality is obvious. The local MHP will be aware of and have links and immediate access to health and social care resources that a regional coordinator will not. Service users, their families and other professionals should have ready access to their care coordinator during times of crisis. Often, the coordinator from the NDMHS is a community mental health nurse (CMHN) who will operate on a 9–5, Monday–Friday basis only. Having cohesive links with local teams is essential should a crisis occur outside working hours, but the ideal is that the deaf person has access to local teams at *all* times.

In the past, it was often the case that referrals to NDMHS were made by lone professionals in local mental health or social work teams. CPA would not be in place at the point of referral and the coordinator role would fall to the first MHP that the deaf person met. The referrer, happy that the deaf service user is receiving input from NDMHS, then closes the case. This can leave the deaf specialist MHP coordinating the care package in isolation and at a distance.

Interestingly, by definition, the involvement of a single professional should place the deaf person under the criteria for **standard** CPA. Yet it has been suggested that the complexities of working with deaf people always require an enhanced approach, regardless of the severity of their mental health problem (DH, 2005). This is both discriminatory to the deaf person and clouds the process in ambiguity.

On a practical level, the basic documentation for regional CPA is different from that of the local CMHT. There is no standardised format for CPA and the level of detail can often reflect this. The accessibility of the care plan is an obvious issue should it be needed quickly. Electronic copies, in keeping with DH recommendations, must be available so that they can be accessed in times of crisis. Incompatibility between regional and local systems can only serve to confuse and fragment care.

Reviewing the Care Package

The specialist deaf service MHP is spread thin geographically. Organising CPA reviews is a notoriously haphazard affair at the best of times. The review of CPA packages organised by NDMHS (in the absence of the committed involvement of local mental health services) tends to comprise the professionals that were involved prior to referral, namely the social worker for the deaf, the service user and their carers. The author has known a GP fail to attend a CPA review even when it was held at **their own** practice.

For in-patient services, the attendance of local care professionals for CPA reviews is inconsistent depending upon a number of variables, including distance and availability. The upshot is a process that fails to measure up to guidance.

SUGGESTIONS FOR IMPROVING THE CPA IMPLEMENTATION

It makes basic sense for the NDMHS to work as a tertiary service in keeping with its design and resources. This premise has been acknowledged at a macro level (DH, 2005). In reality the NDMHS is treated as a secondary service when most agencies refer service users. From this point on, the CPA process becomes compromised for deaf service users and the MHP attempting to meet their needs. Redressing the strategic imbalance is vital if deaf people are to receive equitable mental health services.

SINGLE POINT OF ENTRY REFERRAL PROCESS

It is the author's opinion that CPA implementation would improve if there were change in the process of referral, and that the use of 'gateway workers' would facilitate this. The role of the gateway worker is to:

> strengthen access, and to provide community triage for people who may need urgent contact with specialist mental health services. (DH, 2002, p. 4)

The gateway worker bridges systematic gaps in the current referral process. This is enhanced by remits within GP and primary-care teams. From this position, the gateway worker should be able to coordinate care plans at a local level, thus improving access for deaf people needing various levels of mental health service.

The pathway illustrated in Figure 15.3 promotes equal access for deaf service users and encourages more systematic and collaborative applications of CPA. As with hearing people, this process facilitates a single entry point for the deaf person to access services. After being seen by the GP, the deaf person will be referred to the gateway worker for assessment. The gateway worker must have sufficient Deaf awareness, skills and knowledge to ensure accurate assessment. The DH has pledged its commitment and has made local services aware of their responsibilities in providing appropriate levels of skill to meet the needs of its Deaf community (DH, 2005).

If the assessment identifies the deaf person as being suitable for input at primary-care level, the implementation of CPA is not relevant, for example if the person requires anxiety management or assertiveness-skills training. However, if the persons needs appear more complex or enduring, the deaf person will be signposted to the local secondary care level: CMHT. It will then be the responsibility of the CMHT to conduct a mental health assessment, allot the appropriate level of CPA and allocate a local care coordinator. The CMHT again need to have individuals in place who have the appropriate skills to facilitate the assessment of a person who is deaf. Should the assessment prove problematic or the outcomes suggest treatment strategies not available locally (psychotherapy, psychological assessment or specialist occupational therapy as case examples), this would be an appropriate point to refer the service user to the NDMHS. If the deaf person requires admission to hospital for a short time, the option is open for an in-patient stay within the NDMHS.

The important factor is that the referral will have been generated by the CPA process and taken forward by an existing care coordinator at a local level. This person will remain involved, working in partnership with the NDMHS and, as coordinator, retain overall responsibility for a member of the local community. It is the responsibility of the local team to implement recommendations made by the NDMHS following the assessment. The NDMHS would offer support and guidance to localities to ensure that implementation is effective and adequately meeting the needs of the deaf person.

There is an expectation that the focus of local primary care and the CMHT will be upon the needs of their Deaf communities (DH, 2005). The effectiveness of the deaf mental health pathway is dependent upon a firm commitment to existing philosophies laid down by the DH. This means positively encouraging those MHPs with an active interest in working with members of the Deaf community and rewarding those for their work in such a valuable role.

THE RECOVERY PARADIGM: DEFINITION AND HISTORY

Recovery is concerned with establishing an evidence-based ethos that is contrary to the traditional approaches to the care of the mentally ill (Harding and Zahnister, 1994; De Girolamo, 1996). It gives the service user a sense of future using coping strategies, not the false promise of a cure (Deegan, 2001). As a concept, recovery is unique in that it is the only paradigm that has been perpetuated by active demands of the client group it duly serves (Turner and Frak, 2001). Rising from the ashes of the civil rights movements of the sixties, the user/survivor advocates challenged the concept of mental illness as a prerequisite for social exclusion (Carling, 1995). As such, societal views of mental health have been inadvertently reinforced by those who are employed to 'care for' service users.

Szasz (1989) notes that such disparity is a reflection of a system devised around public protection, with stigma as the natural upshot. To address this imbalance, social exclusion and stigma are a focal point for recovery approaches since such facets reinforce mental illness as a

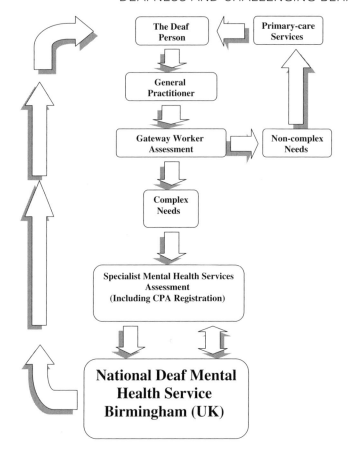

Figure 15.2 Suggested referral process framework

disease from which the sufferer has no hope of living a fulfilled life (DH, 2004).

Relevance to CPA

There is an expectation that care coordinators consider a recovery-based ethos when working with the service user to formulate the CPA care plan (DH, 1999a). However, in its agenda to provide a systematic approach, CPA has been criticised for compromising client-centred perspectives.

Stickley and Masterson (2003) argue that any acknowledgement of the service user's subjective or lived experience is either negated or rendered irrelevant by the CPA's fundamental philosophy of risk assessment, risk management and protection of the public. This suggests the need for innovative changes in the methods MHPs employ when using the CPA framework in practice.

Failing to do this has the potential to undermine core principles of individualised care identified by Stickley and Masterson as:

> strengths, wishes, desires, interests and hopes (Stickley and Masterson, 2003, p. 26)

The notion of instilling hope within the service user is fundamental to the recovery paradigm (Deegan, 2001). Wierzbicka (1999) suggests that, as a concept, hope is equated with a sense of future good, making it somewhat distanced from the here and now. This separation has obvious implications for service users who are experiencing current crisis, especially considering its abstract nature. It can be argued that recovery-based approaches are viable tools in the delivery of cultural cogence and the notion of service user empowerment within the existing CPA framework.

Relevance to Deaf Service Users and CB

There is an unprecedented parity between the experiences of those who endure SMI and members of the deaf community, for example in the areas of social exclusion and overreliance on the medical perspective (Davis, 1995; Meadow-Orlans and Erting, 2000). Societal values are ascribed to the deaf person as having a disability and it has been established that this dynamic has the long-term propensity to foster dependence, subsequently disempowering the individual (Davis, 1995).

It is acknowledged that frustration and loss of power are key dynamics in the escalation of anger and challenging behaviour (Emerson, 1995). For deaf people, this is no less an issue, considering the traditional sense of cultural oppression and the frustration the Deaf community experiences at the hands of the hearing world (Lane *et al.*, 1996). It becomes readily apparent that creating an environment that reasserts the service user's sense of control will ultimately impact upon subsequent behaviours generated by feelings of powerlessness (National Institute for Clinical Excellence, 2005).

In accepting that there is a notorious power imbalance within the therapeutic relationship, practitioners have traditionally found moral and ethical dilemmas when trying to redress the balance (Grant, 2003). This centres upon the inherent conflict within the role of the MHP as an advocate for individuals that use mental health services and the requirements of public protection enshrined within professional codes and statutory obligations (Marangos-Frost and Wells, 2000). If it is true that the recovery ethic is negated by the risk-assessment/risk-management facets of CPA, any inflexibility within legislative tools will need to be supported with other mechanisms. Given their propensity to promote empowerment, recovery-based frameworks may fit the bill, giving the service user a greater sense of control.

THE WELLNESS AND RECOVERY ACTION PLAN (WRAP)

The idea that hopelessness inhibits recovery and perpetuates crisis is well documented (Deegan, 2001; Barker and Buchanan-Barker, 2004). Exponents of recovery argue that the practitioner must demonstrate a sense of belief that the service user will recover from their current state of crisis while developing skills to manage in the future. Frameworks that encourage individuals to use coping strategies to develop proactive responses during times of crisis have a better chance of averting relapse and becoming hospitalised (Brimblecombe *et al.*, 2003).

The *Wellness and Recovery Action Plan* (Copeland, 2002) is a recovery-based approach that empowers service users by using their own fundamental coping strategies to develop a framework that becomes by definition individual to the person designing it. The MHP facilitates the process of completing the tool but the service user is the true author, incorporating aspects of their lived experience to inform the content. In so doing, the MHP can remain an advocate for the person and not impact upon the therapeutic alliance (Grant, 2003).

Copeland defines the WRAP programme as a:

> structured system for monitoring uncomfortable and distressing symptoms and, through planned responses, reducing, modifying or eliminating those symptoms (Copeland, 2002, p. 3)

The WRAP is divided into six sections that encourage the person to devise their own daily maintenance plan (DMP) and use self-management strategies to manage relapse and crisis. As the format consists of a series of lists, this could be readily transferred into British

Part 1	Part 2	Part 3	Part 4	Part 5	Part 6
Wellness Tool Box	DMP	Triggers	Early Warning Signs	When Things Are Breaking Down	Crisis Planning

Figure 15.3 Overview of the WRAP framework (adapted from Copeland, 2002)

Sign Language (BSL) and/or pictorial representation. Figure 15.3 offers an overview of the WRAP framework.

Coupled to this is the person's post-crisis plan, which supports the individual during the initial stages of crisis recovery. This plan is more flexible than the framework above in that:

it is constantly changing as you heal (Copeland, 2002, p. 41)

The overall feel of the WRAP is that it is very much service-user focused and led. In keeping with national guidance for the use of advanced directives in crisis planning (DH, 2004), the framework allows for MHPs to have complete knowledge of the wants and needs of the service users for whom they provide a service, based on previous or current experiences.

CONCLUSION

CPA was developed as a means to improve the consistency and delivery of mental healthcare provision in the UK, yet implementation has often reflected the inconsistencies it sought to cure. This has influenced the attitudes of local CMHTs to CPA when deaf people attempt to gain access to services.

The referral process suggested within this chapter is reliant upon a change of such attitudes. It involves local services acknowledging their responsibilities to **all** members of their community. It is unacceptable for local CMHTs, given the DH mandate for equal access to deaf service users, to place these responsibilities upon outside agencies or service providers. Although there should be an expectation that these deaf service providers assist and support local teams.

It has been established that recovery-based ideologies are part of the fabric of current mental health policy and clinical guidance. The pressures upon clinicians to balance statutory obligations and professional advocacy for the service user may be made easier by employing the recovery paradigm. It has value as a mechanism to stabilise the therapeutic alliance, which is all too often under threat from the rigid application of mental healthcare systems.

The frameworks suggested here are a source for much-needed debate. The search for more effective interregional working can only offer hope for deaf service users and their families. As practitioners and service providers, it is a debate that we are obligated to perpetuate and resolve.

REFERENCES

Anthony P, Crawford P (2000) Service user involvement in care planning: the mental health nurse's perspective. *Journal of Psychiatric and Mental Health Nursing* 7(5): 425–34.

Audit Commission (1986) *Making a Reality of Community Care*, London, HMSO.

Audit Commission (1994) *Finding a Place: A Review of Mental Health Services for Adults*, London, HMSO.

Barker P, Buchanan-Barker P (2004) Beyond empowerment: revering the story-teller. *Mental Health Practice* 7(5): 18–20.

Barre T, Evans R (2005) Integration: holy writ or shibboleth? *Mental Health Practice* 3(9): 40–3.

Brimblecombe N, O'Sullivan G, Parkinson B (2003) Home treatment as an alternative to inpatient admission: characteristics of those treated and factors predicting hospitalization. *Journal of Psychiatric and Mental Health Nursing* 10(6): 683–7.

Carling PJ (1995) *Return to the Community: Building Support Systems for People with Psychiatric Disabilities*, New York, Guilford Press.

Coleman R (1999) *Recovery: An Alien Concept*, Gloucester, Handsell.

Copeland ME (2002) *Wellness and Recovery Action Plan*, West Dummerston, Peach Press.

Davis LJ (1995) *Enforcing Normalcy: Disability, Deafness and the Body*, New York, Verso Books.

Deegan PE (2001) Recovery as a self-directed process of healing and transformation. In Brown C (ed), *Recovery and Wellness: Models of Hope and Empowerment for People with Mental Illness*, New York, Haworth Press.

De Girolamo G (1996) WHO studies on schizophrenia: an overview of the results and their implications for the understanding of the disorder. *The Psychotherapy Patient* 9(3–4): 213–23.

Department of Health (1990a) *The NHS and Community Care Act*, London, HMSO.

Department of Health (1990b) *Caring for People: The Care Programme Approach for People with a Mental Illness Referred to Specialist Mental Health Services*, joint Health/Social Services Circular: C (90) 23/LASS (90)11 London, DOH.

Department of Health (1990c) *Community Care in the Next Decade and Beyond: Policy Guidance*, London, HMSO.

Department of Health (1995) *Building Bridges: A Guide to Arrangements for Inter-agency Working for the Care and Protection of Severely Mentally Ill People*, London, HMSO.

Department of Health (1997) *The New NHS: Modern, Dependable*, London, TSO.

Department of Health (1998) *A First Class Service: Quality in the New NHS*, London, TSO.

Department of Health (1999a) *Effective Care Co-ordination in Mental Health Services: Modernizing the Care Programme Approach: A Policy Booklet*, London, TSO.

Department of Health (1999b) *National Service Framework for Mental Health*, London, TSO.

Department of Health (2002) *A Sign of the Times: Modernising Mental Health Services for People Who are Deaf*, London, Department of Health.

Department of Health (2004) *From Here to Equality: A Strategic Plan to Tackle Stigma and Discrimination on Mental Health Grounds*, Leeds, NIMHE.

Department of Health (2005) *Mental Health and Deafness: Towards Equity and Access*, London, TSO.

Department of Health and Social Security (1988) *Report of the Committee of Inquiry into the Care and After Care of Sharon Campbell*, (Chairman: J. Spokes), London, HMSO.

Department of Health and Social Security (1989) *Caring for People: Community Care in the Next Decade and Beyond*, London, HMSO.

Department of Health and Welsh Office (1999) *Code of Practice: Mental Health Act* (1983), London, TSO.

Emerson E (2001) *Challenging Behaviour: Analysis and Intervention in People with Severe Intellectual Disabilities* (2nd edn.), Cambridge, Cambridge University Press.

Grant A (2003) Freedom and consent. In Barker P (ed), *Psychiatric and Mental Health Nursing: the Craft of Caring*, London, Arnold, pp. 522–31.

Griffiths R (1988) *Community Care: Agenda for Action*, London, HMSO.

Harding CM, Zahnister JH (1994) Empirical correction of seven myths about schizophrenia with implications for treatment. *Acta Psychiatrica Scandanavica* 90(384): 140–6.

Health and Safety Executive (2003) *Five Steps to Risk Assessment*, London, HSE.

Lane H, Hoffmeister R, Bahan B (1996) *A Journey into the Deaf-World*, San Diego, Dawn Sign Press.

Marangos-Frost S, Wells D (2000) Psychiatric nurses' thoughts and feelings about restraint use: a decision dilemma. *Journal of Advanced Nursing* 31(2): 362–9.

May P (1996) Joint training for mental health key workers: Part 1. *Nursing Standard* 10(43): 39–42.

McDermott G (1998) The care programme approach: a patient perspective. *Nursing Times* 94(8): 57–9.

Meadow-Orlans K, Erting C (2000) Deaf people in society. In Hindley P, Kitson N (eds), *Mental Health and Deafness*, London, Whurr, pp. 3–24.

Miller C, Freeman M, Ross N (2001) *Inter-Professional Practice in Health and Social Care: Challenging the Shared Learning Agenda*, London, Arnold.

Mishcon J, Sensky T, Lindsey M, Cook S (2000) *Report of the Independent Inquiry Team into the Care and Treatment of Daniel Joseph*, London, Merton Sutton and Wandsworth Health Authority and Lambeth, Southwark and Lewisham Health Authority.

Mueser KT, Bond GR, Drake RE, Resnick SG (1998) Models of community care for severe mental illness: a review of research on case management. *Schizophrenia Bulletin* 24(1): 37–74.

National Institute for Clinical Excellence (2005) *The Short-term Management of Disturbed/Violent Behaviour in In-patient Psychiatric Settings and Emergency Departments*, London, TSO.

Peck E, Norman I (1999) Working together in adult community mental health services: exploring inter-professional role relations. *Journal of Mental Health* 8(3): 231–42.

Peoples K (2002) Ethical challenges in training professionals for mental health services with deaf people. In Gutman V (ed), *Ethics in Mental Health and Deafness*, Washington, Gallaudet University Press, pp. 99–122.

Pollard RQ (2002) Ethical conduct in research involving deaf people. In Gutman V (ed), *Ethics in Mental Health and Deafness*, Washington Gallaudet University Press, pp. 162–78.

Ritchie S (1994) *Report of the Inquiry into the Care and Treatment of Christopher Clunis*, London, HMSO.

Rush B (2004) Mental health service user involvement in England: lessons from history. *Journal of Psychiatric and Mental Health Nursing* 11(3) 313–18.

Shepherd D (1996) *Learning the Lessons: Mental Health Inquiry Reports Published in England and Wales Between 1969 and 1996 and their Recommendations for Improving Practice* (2nd edn.), London, Zito Trust.

Simpson A, Miller C, Bowers L (2003) The history of the care programme approach England: where did it go wrong? *Journal of Mental Health* 12(5): 489–504.

Stickley T, Masterson S (2003) An uncaring approach? *Mental Health Today* March: 24–6.

Szasz T (1989) *Law, Liberty and Psychiatry*, New York, Syracuse University Press.

Turner D, Frak D (2001) *Wild Geese: A Report on a Six Month Consultancy on the Recovery Approach*, London, National Schizophrenia Fellowship.

Wallace M (1986) A caring community? The plight of Britain's mentally ill. *Sunday Times Magazine* (3 May), pp. 25–38.

Warner L (2005) *Review of the Literature on the Care Programme Approach*, London, The Sainsbury Centre for Mental Health.

Wierzbicka A (1999) *Emotions Across Languages and Cultures: Diversity and Universals*, New York, Cambridge University Press.

PART IV
Forensic Services

16

Deaf People and the Criminal Justice System

SUE O'ROURKE AND REBECCA REED

INTRODUCTION

The little that has been written about deaf people in the criminal justice system consists of anecdotal accounts about deaf people being in a disadvantageous position in relation to their hearing peers due to concerns of language and deprivation. In this chapter, the prevention of genuine participation in the process of law by discriminatory practices within the system is highlighted. The apparent insufficient understanding that many deaf people exhibit in court is discussed with particular reference to the issue of fitness to plead. It is argued that difficulties in understanding the criminal justice procedures may be more a factor of culture and language than of the ability of the deaf person.

Historically, deaf people have been viewed as incompetent. These perceptions have their origin in the argument that in order to think we need language. Since speech is equated with language, those who cannot speak are deemed incapable of thought (Lane, 1984). The logic of this argument is obviously flawed, since sign language is indeed a language in the absence of speech. However, although the premise may no longer be explicitly accepted, the assumption of incompetence still exists in many people's attitudes and can be found frequently in a legal context.

Deafness and Challenging Behaviour: The 360° Perspective. Edited by S. Austen and D. Jeffery
© 2007 John Wiley & Sons Ltd

DEAF CULTURE, HEARING CULTURE AND LEGAL CULTURE

Deaf culture is described elsewhere and will not be examined in detail here. But there are situations where cultures clash, and there is a distinct misunderstanding. Fox (2005) describes many humorous and not-so-humorous encounters between English people and those from other countries. Many difficulties arise due to the English tendency to avoid directness and to talk around a subject without getting to the point. In fact, this 'Englishness' could equally be called 'English hearing culture' and is observed by deaf people to be a very strange set of rules indeed. Deaf colleagues have frequently observed how hearing colleagues rarely say what they mean and take an age to get to the point. Conversely, deaf people (or hearing people absorbed in deaf culture and forgetting the hearing/English rules!) are often seen as too blunt and, as a result, socially unskilled. Deaf people need to know they are not alone in finding hearing/English culture odd and difficult to fathom.

If all this applies in day-to-day encounters, how much more so does it exist in the ritualistic and jargon-laden world of the criminal justice system? Deaf people encountering the police, lawyers, courts and prison system find themselves in a situation where few people have awareness of deaf issues; the language used is often complex and abstract and involves concepts out of their experience, and which are difficult to understand.

DEAF PEOPLE AND THE POLICE

There is a lack of research concerning the interaction between the police and deaf people. The literature consists mainly of articles expressing concern about accessibility to police services. For example, a recent meeting between deaf people in an area of Manchester focused on difficulty accessing services out of hours, which are currently only available by telephone, the suggestion that digital signs are used in the police station to help give instructions and the recommendation that reception staff learn some basic British Sign Language (BSL) (Trafford Today, 2005). It is somewhat disheartening that such simple matters are still being discussed, and does not bode well for consideration of more complex issues such as how deaf people who are arrested participate in police interviews or understand their rights.

The Police and Criminal Evidence Act 1984 (PACE HMSO, 1984) states that if, on arrest, the custody officer suspects that a person may be deaf they are required to contact a sign language interpreter as soon as possible. Code C of the Code of Conduct relating to the Act suggests that if a person is suspected to be mentally disordered or otherwise mentally vulnerable then there must be an 'appropriate adult' present at the interview. This could be a relative or carer, someone experienced in working with mentally vulnerable individuals who is not a police officer, or another responsible adult aged 18 or over who is not employed by the police. The Act explains that the role of the appropriate adult is to:

- advise the interviewee
- observe whether the interview is being conducted properly and fairly
- facilitate communication.

In the opinion of the authors, in the case of a deaf person, in order to perform this role adequately the appropriate adult must be a fluent sign language user, which frequently is not the case. Although the first task of the appropriate adult, to advise the interviewee, may be carried out via an interpreter, the second and third require access to both the English form of questioning and BSL, since a major aspect of the proper conduct of the interview is the accurate interpretation of English into BSL and vice versa.

Interviews by the police are routinely audiotaped. In certain circumstances, they may be visually recorded also. The PACE *Code of Conduct* suggests that this **might** be appropriate in cases where the interviewee is deaf or deaf/blind or speech-impaired and uses sign language to communicate. In the absence of training within the police force in relation to deaf awareness, this begs the question as to how a police officer would be equipped to decide whether a deaf person would be vulnerable and require their interview to be visually recorded. The *Code of Conduct* also says that it might be appropriate to use visual recording in cases where an appropriate adult is required. However, it also states that there may be authorisation not to visually record an interview where it is not reasonably practical to do so and rectifying this would delay the interview. The result of this is that many interviews with deaf people in police custody are undertaken without visual recording and an audio recording of the English interpretation of BSL is made and then transcribed. This puts the interpreter in a vulnerable position as he/she can later be challenged on the interpretation and there is no record of the original. More importantly, the only record is that of the words chosen by the interpreter. In any given situation, the interpreter has to make numerous choices about the exact words to use, and these may not always be a fair representation of what the deaf person said. Without recourse to viewing a visual recording, there is no means of challenging the interpretation, therefore rendering the deaf interviewee vulnerable.

DEAF PEOPLE IN COURT

The position of deaf people in court has received scant attention in the literature. There are guidelines published about support needed in court such as interpreters, but little in the way of empirical research. One exception to this is the excellent study by Brennan and Brown (1997). This looks at the role of interpreters in court, making observations of what happened to language in that setting and the impact of this. The results are startling and highlight the mismatch between the legal setting and the needs of deaf people. In particular, the study illustrates the mismatch between the use of language in a legal setting and the naturalistic use of BSL. For example, it was frequently observed that open-ended questions were changed in the interpretation to multiple-choice questions, thus limiting the possible responses available to the deaf person and possibly leading them without the knowledge of the court. Descriptions of court proceedings show how interpreters have to make a raft of choices in changing what is said from a verbal to a visual language, and in doing so may add extraneous information. For example, if the question was: 'Did you proceed down the corridor?', the interpreter will show in BSL where the corridor was in relation to the person and the manner of 'proceeding' (e.g. whether walking or running). This is all information that has to be chosen by the interpreter without prior knowledge and without the awareness of the court. This process can affect witness responses and how the case proceeds.

In court, it is necessary to be able to understand BSL and English in order to fully appreciate the changes in language that need to take place to facilitate understanding. The study by Brennan and Brown (1997) shows that interpreted BSL is often very far from the original English, without the knowledge of the court.

Although the focus of the study is on the accuracy of translation, the results also point to a raft of psychological factors that mean the deaf person is at risk of being placed at a disadvantage in the courtroom. These include the psychological concepts of acquiescence, compliance and suggestibility, which are discussed below.

'FITNESS TO PLEAD'

Deaf people, or rather one deaf person in particular, has been crucial in shaping legal process in relation to fitness to plead. Glen Pearson, a young deaf man of limited intellectual ability and with minimal language skills, was accused of a minor acquisitive offence. He was found unfit to plead, by virtue of learning disability and communicative incompetence. At the time, being unfit to plead automatically meant a disposal at a high secure hospital, in this case Rampton Hospital in Nottinghamshire. Acknowledging the ludicrously disproportionate outcome in this case, he was discharged shortly afterwards by a mental health review tribunal. This case was influential in changing the law in 1991 to allow for a 'trial of the facts'. In situations where the defendant is found unfit to plead, and the case is sufficiently serious to be in the public interest to pursue, a trial of the facts can conclude that in all likelihood the person did commit the offence, although the burden of proof is on the balance of probability only. In this instance, a range of disposals are now possible commensurate with the person's needs. Whereas in the past the only option available to the court was to send the person to a high secure hospital, now there may be admission to a variety of hospital settings in varying degrees of security, according to the risk posed by the individual or even a treatment order in the community.

When a deaf person finds themselves in court, frequently their lawyer or the court requests an assessment for fitness to plead. In a study by Young *et al.* (2001), it was found that a high proportion of the forensic referrals received by a specialist mental health service requested an opinion on whether an individual was fit to plead or fit to stand trial. The frequency of such requests may reflect the assumption of incompetence discussed earlier, or an acknowledgement that deaf people may be vulnerable in the criminal justice system.

In order to be 'fit', a defendant has to understand the charges against her/him, be able to instruct a lawyer, understand the function of the court, judge, barristers and jury. He or she also has to be able to understand the right to object to a jury. Individuals, deaf or hearing, can have difficulty with this for a variety of reasons. A person with a mental illness may be found temporarily unfit to plead as her/his active symptoms of psychosis prevent understanding of proceedings. In this instance, the person may require treatment and then be returned to court at a time when he or she is then judged to be fit to plead. People with a learning disability or acquired brain injury may be unfit to plead due to intellectual impairment, depending on the extent of impairment and the nature of the case. Fitness has to be related to the complexity of the case and the charges, as more complex issues are more difficult to understand.

INTELLECTUAL IMPAIRMENT AND FITNESS TO PLEAD

If a defendant is assessed to have an IQ under 70, it is highly likely that he or she will be found unfit to plead by virtue of 'mental impairment', the term used in the Mental Health Act 1983. Deaf or hearing defendants may be unfit to plead due to mental impairment. Assessment using appropriate non-verbal measures of intellectual ability, administered by a specialist clinical psychologist using BSL, can ascertain whether a person has a learning disability. This is usually achieved using the performance subtests of the Wechsler Adult Intelligence Scale, currently in its third edition (WAIS III, Wechsler, 1997). Such non-verbal measures have been shown to produce a reliable and valid indication of intellectual capacity in deaf people (Braden, 1994). However, although non-verbal abilities are required in order to complete the task, a certain degree of linguistic competence is required to understand task instructions. Thus, in individuals with minimal language skills, this can be problematic and there is a danger of underestimating non-verbal cognitive ability simply because the individual did not understand the task. Having said this, pragmatically speaking, if a person cannot understand the instruction in BSL, 'Tell me what is missing?' (from the Picture Completion subtest of the WAIS-III), they are unlikely to understand court proceedings.

If testing shows there is intellectual impairment, the task then is to consider whether the impairment is sufficient to preclude understanding of the proceedings in relation to a particular offence. In cases where the scores fall in the learning disability range (performance IQ < 70), this is almost always the case, especially since non-verbal IQ is best seen as a measure of capacity or potential, and most deaf people function at a lower level in terms of acquired knowledge due to barriers in accessing information. In cases where IQ is above 70, considering fitness to plead can be more complicated, as the issue is often one of deprivation rather than disability.

DEPRIVATION AND FITNESS TO PLEAD

Difficulties arise when the individual concerned tests as 'within normal limits' on non-verbal tests of intellectual ability but, for reasons of deprivation, clearly has little understanding and can be considered unfit to plead. In this case, there is a discrepancy between intellectual capacity and attainment of knowledge, skills and information to a degree that is rarely seen in hearing people. A hearing person, growing up in disadvantaged circumstances may skip school, have few positive role models and grow up not achieving educationally or socially. Very occasionally, there are cases of hearing feral children, or those subject to extreme abuse and cut off from normal interaction. However, for deaf people growing up in situations with no access to an effective means of communication, this means that the deprivation in all areas is profound. Communication is the route of access to all knowledge; to deprive a deaf child of a means of communicating affects all areas of development and, in particular, affects social and emotional development. Those deaf adults who have grown up in exclusively hearing environments, who may have been treated as disabled and incompetent, who have had poor educational experiences in a setting which has left them baffled and who have no chance of acquiring information incidentally are seriously disadvantaged. Such deprivation can lead to what is commonly called 'minimal language skills', and is often seen in cases where exposure to sign language has only occurred late in childhood or even as a young adult. There are other deaf people who have suffered an impoverished childhood albeit less dramatically than some of their peers. Growing up in a hearing family with no sign language and attending an oral school in which they struggle can lead to deprivation of learning, both formal and incidental, which impacts on adult adjustment. These deaf individuals are disadvantaged by virtue of the amount of information they have missed as a child developing in a non-communicating environment. They are likely to find the concepts involved in court proceedings very difficult to understand, as if the new knowledge that they must acquire in this new setting has nothing to latch on to.

The courts in the United Kingdom find this presentation very difficult to cope with. While a person with a history of deprivation may clearly not be able to understand and is obviously not fit to plead, they are neither mentally ill nor mentally impaired, in the sense of having a learning disability. In fact, their intellectual potential is within normal limits. Functional impairment borne out of linguistic deprivation poses a dilemma to the courts in the UK and the USA (Vernon *et al.*, 2000). In the UK, the court may accept that the deaf person with minimal language skills and a history of deprivation is unable to understand proceedings and is thus unfit to plead. In this case, a trial of the facts may proceed with the possibility of a range of disposals, as discussed above. However, the court may also find that, in the absence of a formal mental illness or impairment, the person is fit to plead despite the assessment of experts that this is not the case.

Case Study One

A deaf woman in her thirties was in court in relation to an assault charge. She had appeared evasive in police interviews and this was interpreted as her not wishing to answer questions. Her solicitor was concerned that she did not follow the questions and asked for a psychological opinion as to her level of understanding. She tested in the low–average range on non-verbal tests of intellectual ability. However, her history was of being brought up in an oral school and of struggling to understand her teachers and her family. It was suggested that deprivation during development had impaired her understanding. In particular, she had difficulty in answering general questions, tending instead to reply with specific examples. In addition, she struggled to talk about instances outside her own experience or comment on possibilities. The court accepted her difficulties and, although she was deemed to have capacity, accommodated her by having the psychologist monitor the proceedings and check understanding at regular breaks throughout the hearing.

VULNERABILITY IN COURT

Prominent miscarriages of justice have attracted media attention over recent years. It is now accepted that vulnerable individuals may be disadvantaged by court proceedings and make false confessions, or be led by cross-examination to incriminate themselves. Research has shown that certain groups of people are more likely to be vulnerable than others and certain characteristics of interrogation or cross-examination can lead to increased vulnerability. In these circumstances, it can be demonstrated that vulnerable witnesses and defendants have a tendency towards acquiescence, compliance or suggestibility.

ACQUIESCENCE

Acquiescence is the tendency to answer in the affirmative any question that is asked; the most frequently observed being the tendency to nod when asked, 'Do you understand?' This may be in order to please the person asking the question, to avoid looking incompetent by owning up to not understanding or to achieve some goal, such as being allowed to leave as quickly as possible. The tendency to acquiesce can be assessed by observation only, or in a person who says they understand by checking that this is the case. A brief informal assessment may be carried out in which the person is asked whether they agree with a series of statements, half of which are in opposition to the others, for example, 'Do you think the Prime Minister is doing a good job?' and 'Do you think the Prime Minister is useless?' If the answer 'yes' is given to over 50% of the questions, it can be concluded that the person tends towards an acquiescent response. Of course, this a somewhat simplistic assessment, since the person is more likely to be 'vulnerable' if the questions are difficult to understand or beyond their experience. This may create an anxiety response that in turn makes it difficult for the person to say they do not understand. In order to save face, they give an acquiescent response.

COMPLIANCE

Compliance is the tendency to agree to a proposition to achieve some gain. For example, a person under arrest may sign a confession simply in order to be let out of the police station, while being fully aware that he or she did not commit the crime. Thus, compliance does not involve internal acceptance of the proposition. Gudjonsson (1989) has developed a compliance questionnaire. However, this is not appropriate for use with deaf people, for linguistic reasons (O'Rourke and Grewer, 2005), and therefore, to date, the only means of assessing compliance in deaf people is by observation.

SUGGESTIBILITY

Suggestibility is the extent to which the individual comes to accept the proposition within the question as true, in other words the extent to which the person can be led in her or his responses by the characteristic of the interrogation. In this case, there is internal acceptance of the proposition, in contrast to compliance. An example, given in Figure 16.1,

Leading question	Non-suggestible response	Suggestible response
'Did you go to the house in the morning or the afternoon?'	'I didn't go to the house.'	'In the morning.'
'Did you have a knife or a gun?'	'Neither.'	'I didn't have a gun' (implying a knife).

Figure 16.1 Examples of suggestible responses

will illustrate how a suggestible person might respond to leading questions, compared to someone who is not suggestible.

Characteristics of the individual, the setting and the interrogator have been shown to relate to suggestibility. Broadly speaking, a person is more likely to be suggestible if he or she is less knowledgeable, less powerful and more anxious (Gudjonsson, 1991). The setting can provoke a suggestible response by being more intimidating, and emphasising the power differential between the individual being questioned and the interrogator. It is difficult to find a situation that might meet these criteria more fully than the one of a deaf person in a court.

Given the findings in relation to suggestibility, it seems reasonable to propose that deaf people might be more suggestible than hearing people. The only study to investigate this using standard measures of suggestibility (O'Rourke and Beail, 2004) found that, when given access to information via BSL, deaf people are not, in fact, more suggestible than their hearing peers. However, it is suggested that in real-life situations where access to the event that the person is being questioned about is likely to be limited, and questioning is not likely to be deaf-friendly, the risk of suggestibility remains. It is recommended that more ecologically valid investigations in this area be carried out in the future.

EQUALITY OF ACCESS TO THE CRIMINAL JUSTICE SYSTEM

DEAF JURORS

Currently, deaf people in the UK are not permitted to sit on a jury. There is considerable controversy over this issue. The view of deaf charities and human rights advisers is that deaf people should have the same rights and responsibilities as hearing people. However, the courts hold the view that it is not in the best interest of the defendant to have a juror who cannot 'hear the evidence' (Winter, 1980). Current law in England states that a thirteenth person is not allowed in the jury room while deliberations are taking place. This precludes deaf people from taking part in jury service, as an interpreter would be a thirteenth person. In the United States, deaf people are able to serve as jurors. Judges have ruled that it would be illegal to exclude a person from jury service solely on the grounds of their disability. Interpreters accompany the deaf person to court, and in their interpretation try to show exactly how the defendant spoke, whether they appeared scared, were loud or spoke very quietly. Judges and attorneys admit that deaf jurors often pick up on observations that their hearing counterparts would not (Kumar, 2000). However, there are still critics of the system in the US with some attorneys arguing that their client's ability to have a fair trial should outweigh the deaf person's right to carry out jury service, although the way in which a deaf person makes it 'unfair' is not clear (Winter, 1980).

DEAF VICTIMS AND WITNESSES

It goes without saying that deaf people who use BSL require a sign language interpreter in police interviews and in court. There are individual interpreters and interpreting companies who specialise in this area of work. They tend to work as a team of three in court, so at any one time there is one person interpreting, a second monitoring and assisting, while the third person has a break. In this way there is monitoring of accuracy to some extent. Specialist interpreters have the advantage of being familiar with the court setting and some of the legal jargon, and have the confidence to interrupt proceedings if necessary, either because the spoken English is too fast or additional time is needed to interpret a concept accurately. In addition, deaf individuals with minimal language skills, impaired cognitive ability or difficulties in understanding due to deprivation may benefit from the employment of a deaf relay. This usually comes about in situations where the interpreters involved in the case make the lawyers or the court aware that the individual concerned is not able to follow proceedings, or else there is prior knowledge about the person's level of functioning, which suggests a relay is needed. The relay is a deaf person who is employed to take the interpreted version and put it into more accessible BSL, at a level the person can understand. This changes the process considerably as the interpreting can no longer be simultaneous but has to be consecutive. This means that information has to be given in chunks, interpreted first to the deaf relay and then communicated to the deaf person. This stop-start method can be difficult for the court to cope with, as lawyers feel the flow of their questioning is interrupted and also adds considerably to the time needed to hear a case.

A major new development in improving the ability of vulnerable people to access the criminal justice system is the establishment of intermediaries. These people are employed by the Home Office and work for the court and have the role of enabling victims and witnesses to understand proceedings and participate more fully. This might involve explaining legal jargon, empowering the person to say when they do not understand or visiting the courtroom to explain the process prior to the hearing commencing. Intermediaries are contacted by the Criminal Prosecution Service or the Police in the event of identifying that a witness is vulnerable and needs support.

The Home Office has initiated a pilot project employing eighty intermediaries in six areas of the country. Included in this is the employment of one deaf intermediary who has a background in working with vulnerable deaf adults and also has worked as a relay. There are plans to roll out the project to other areas of the country in 2007, but no specific plans to increase the number of deaf intermediaries.

DEAF DEFENDANTS

One of the ways access should be improved in the case of deaf defendants is via the use of appropriate adults under PACE. However, as indicated earlier, anecdotal accounts would suggest that often the appropriate adult is unfamiliar with deafness or BSL and therefore unable to perform this role adequately.

There are a number of ways in which the court can become more accessible, so as not to disadvantage deaf defendants, as described above. At present, the intermediary service does not extend to defendants. Yet this role is often what is needed in order that deaf defendants are not seriously disadvantaged in the criminal justice system. The current provision under the Youth Justice and Criminal Evidence Act 1999 (HMSO, 1999) does not allow for their use with defendants. However, it would be possible for a deaf defendant to make an application to a judge to been given the services of an intermediary. Were there to be a ruling by a judge using her or his inherent powers, this would set a precedent and new legislation would be required in order that intermediaries are made available to vulnerable defendants.

ACCESS DOES NOT ALWAYS MEAN UNDERSTANDING

The accommodations for deaf people described above will all improve the likelihood of access to the criminal justice system. However, there are instances when, despite best efforts, the individual is unable to participate fully. The court could be forgiven for thinking that the deaf person has full access judging by the presence of several interpreters and relays. Nevertheless, it is always advisable, if understanding is in doubt, to stop proceedings at regular intervals and check what has been understood, as described in the case example above.

DEAF PEOPLE IN PRISON

PREVALENCE OF DEAF PRISONERS

It is impossible to know how many deaf prisoners there are in the UK, owing to the fact that neither the courts nor the Home Office keep records on the number who have been tried or sentenced. A Home Office survey in 1996 estimated that 0.1% of the prison population have a 'hearing impairment' (HM Prison Service, 1996). These figures need to be viewed with caution as the survey did not distinguish between hearing impairment as an audiological problem and deafness associated with sign language and cultural identity (Young *et al.*, 2000). It has been estimated that in England and Wales, at any one time, there are between 63 and 100 deaf prisoners whose first or preferred language is BSL (Gibbs and Ackerman, 1999).

A point prevalence study carried out by the National Centre for Mental Health and Deafness in Manchester in 1999 involved sending out questionnaires asking for information on all deaf prisoners. Out of 138 prisons, they received 86 replies and identified 51 prisoners who were deaf or hard of hearing. A survey carried out by Birmingham Deaf Prison Project in 2004 had replies from 77 prisons and found 27 profoundly deaf and 233 hard-of-hearing prisoners. The studies carried out, as well as enabling estimates of prevalence, have highlighted some of the difficulties faced by prisons in meeting the needs of deaf prisoners. Whether the results reflect the true prevalence rates is debatable, partly due to the low response rates to questionnaires and partly as a result of the inability to distinguish different types of deafness and deaf prisoner. The questionnaires were returned by a variety of prison staff including prison officers and healthcare staff, and the response rates were low. However, it is clear that the prison system has no strategic system to identify who is deaf, and the staff do not have the awareness and skills to do this, suggesting that the results of such studies must be treated with caution.

Recently, a prison scoping exercise, funded by the Department of Health (DoH), has been carried out (O'Rourke *et al.*, 2005). Questionnaires were sent to all 138 prisons and young offenders institutions in England and Wales. There was an 83% response rate for replies and 135 deaf prisoners identified out of a total prison population of approximately 76 000 (December, 2005). Again, results can only be seen as a rough estimate due to methodological problems in accurate identification of deaf prisoners. Since prisons have no strategy for dealing with deaf prisoners, there is generally no account taken of their needs. At reception into prison, deaf individuals are not identified and even disability and diversity officers will not be aware of a deaf person unless the deaf person presents themselves and declares an unmet need. In addition, the fact that there is no expertise in deafness within the prison system means that staff are not in a position to be aware of the existence of deaf people, let alone meet their needs. Qualitative results from the scoping exercise highlighted these points and illustrated also that, when a deaf person comes to the attention of the prison service, it can be extremely difficult to even meet basic needs, for example get funding for BSL interpreters.

ACCESS IN PRISONS

If prisons do not have the facilities to identify deaf prisoners and there is no strategic planning to meet their needs, it is not surprising that there are difficulties in accessing facilities. One result of this is that deaf prisoners are not able to distract themselves from the difficulties of prison life in the way that their hearing peers might. For example, the prison service survey (HM Prison Service, 1996) it was found that out of 118 establishments none had minicoms (text phones for deaf people) or teletext subtitles.

The lack of deaf awareness amongst prison staff and the fact that very few officers can use sign language inevitably leads to increased isolation. There is evidence that deaf prisoners often are unable to understand even the most basic procedures or even understand why they are in prison (Egan, 1996; Vernon and Miller, 2005). As one ex-prisoner describes:

> I had difficulties following instructions due to not being able to hear them; I could not hear the announcements over the tannoy or prison

officers shouting me. I think Deaf prisoners should be put altogether in prison and staff should learn to sign. I remember staff wanting to learn BSL but they were told it was too expensive and takes too much time. (O'Rourke *et al.*, 2005)

Frequently, hearing prisoners attend educational classes to improve their skills and as a way of coping with prison life. Many deaf people lack educational skills and could benefit from this. Lack of deaf awareness and difficulties acquiring funding for interpreters often mean that deaf prisoners are not able to attend. A deaf prisoner described how he wanted to go to education classes despite not following the teacher:

I could lip-read quite well but the teacher kept turning his back on the class which was hopeless. When I asked him about this they stopped me going to education and I had to stay in my cell. (O'Rourke *et al.*, 2005)

THE MENTAL HEALTH OF DEAF PRISONERS

Lack of activity or access to distraction can impact on mental health. Prison staff have no training in working with deaf people and so are unable to assess or provide treatment for mental health problems in the deaf prison population. The DoH document 'Mental Health and Deafness: Towards Equity and Access' (2005) identifies the need to consider the mental health needs of deaf prisoners who are isolated within the prison population and therefore at greater risk from mental health problems than their hearing peers.

Mental health professionals with experience of assessing deaf prisoners provide examples of undiagnosed mental disorder and exacerbation of emotional distress due to social isolation and deprivation of communication (O'Rourke *et al.*, 2005). The *Prison Scoping Exercise* (O'Rourke *et al.*, 2005) asks respondents how many of the deaf prisoners identified are in need of a mental health assessment. Of the 135 deaf prisoners, only seven (5.4%) were deemed in need of such an assessment. However, in the majority of cases, the person making this judgement would have neither the effective means of communication with the deaf person nor any awareness of mental health issues in deaf people. This therefore casts doubt on the ability of the staff to decide that the deaf person has no such needs.

Vernon and Miller (2005) describe hearing prisoners who have picked up a little sign language being used as interpreters for deaf prisoners. Obviously, this is highly inappropriate in terms of breaching confidentiality but also is likely to lead to the communication of inaccurate information. In the example below, one deaf prisoner who had good speech and lip-reading skills was used as an interpreter for another deaf prisoner.

Case Study Two

Whilst in prison I was often asked to help another deaf prisoner in different situations, for example when he went to see the doctor or in the canteen (prison shop). I was in the role of interpreter for him. No staff in the prison could sign and I had few friends. I had no minicom so I could not phone my friends or family, I had to ask someone to do it for me.

I remember how in one prison I had to help a deaf prisoner who was suicidal. I was woken up at 1 o'clock in the morning to go to talk to him with two prison officers who could do a few signs. I slept all night on the floor in his cell and in the morning acted as interpreter to tell staff how he was doing.

As the deaf person progresses through the prison system, he is seriously disadvantaged in a number of ways. One difficulty is that prisoners tend to be moved fairly frequently. This means that staff may learn some communication skills, only to find the deaf person has moved on. The prisoner then has to educate a whole new team of staff.

Of concern is the fact that deaf people cannot access prison programmes designed to lower risk, such as the Sex Offender Treatment Programme. This means that, unable to demonstrate change, they are unlikely to get parole and therefore will serve more of their sentence than hearing prisoners. The other aspect of this concerns public protection. If the deaf prisoner cannot access prison programmes and risk-reducing interventions, he is presumably more likely to re-offend on release.

FUTURE DEVELOPMENTS IN THE PRISON SYSTEM

There is growing interest in the plight of deaf prisoners. The DoH has acknowledged this in 'Mental Health and Deafness: Towards Equity and Access' (DoH, 2005), and funding has been granted to undertake a prison in-reach project to deaf prisoners. This will involve a team of professionals specialised in mental health and deafness carrying out assessments on a proportion of the deaf people in prison. Results will make individual recommendations about deaf prisoners and so begin to address unmet need. In addition a report to the DoH will make recommendations about strategic planning for deaf people in the prison service.

CONCLUSION

The common theme throughout this exploration of deaf people within the criminal justice system has been one of exclusion. Whether talking about being interviewed in the police station, appearing in court or being in prison, the deaf person finds him- or herself seriously disadvantaged when compared to their hearing peers.

What exists often when a deaf sign language user finds him- or herself in a legal situation is a clash of cultures and language. Despite the use of interpreters or even deaf relays, there can be a huge chasm between what is being said and the understanding of the deaf person. Of great concern is that the legal professionals are oblivious to this, not having access to both languages. An impression of accuracy is created and the court may be reassured by the appearance of understanding given by a multitude of expert interpreters and relays. Yet those with access to both the English original and BSL and a knowledge of the person's background can often see two things: first that what is interpreted to the deaf person is very far from the original question and, secondly, that the deaf person does not fully understand the question or the implication of the question, which would be apparent in English. Until this difficulty is made explicit in police interviews and in court, Deaf people will not have full and fair participation and the legal professionals will not be gaining an accurate understanding of the deaf person.

REFERENCES

Braden JP (1994) *Deafness, Deprivation and IQ*, New York, Plenum.
Brennan M, Brown G (1997) *Equality Before the Law: Deaf People's Access to Justice*, Durham, Deaf Studies Research Unit.
Department of Health (2005) *Mental Health and Deafness: Towards Equity and Access*, London, Department of Health.
Egan D (1996) *Deafness Behind Bars. See Hear!* BBC2 TV programme 8–9 March 1996.

Fox K (2005) *Watching the English*, London, Hodder & Stoughton General.

Gibbs A and Ackerman N (1999) Deaf prisoners: needs, services and training issues. *Prison Service Journal* 22(32): 31–2.

Gudjonsson GH (1989) Compliance in an interrogation situation: a new scale. *Personality and Individual Differences* 10: 535–40.

Gudjonsson GH (1991) *The Psychology of Interrogations: Confessions and Testimony*, Chichester, Wiley.

Her Majesty's Prison Service (1996) *Survey of Provision for the Physically Disabled*, London, HM Prison Service.

HMSO (1983) *Mental Health Act* 1983, London, TSO.

HMSO (1984) Police and Criminal Evidence Act 1984 (Ch 60) http://www. swarb.co.uk/acts/1984PoliceandCriminalEvidenceAct.shtml, accessed 22 April 2006.

HMSO (1999) Youth Justice and Criminal Evidence Act 1999, http://www. opsi.gov.uk/acts/acts1999/19990023.htm, accessed 24 June 2006.

Kumar A (2000) Deafness is no obstacle for jury duty in bay area. *St Petersburg Times*, 5 June 2000.

Lane H (1984) *When the Mind Hears: A History of the Deaf*, New York, Random House.

O'Rourke S, Beail N (2004) Suggestibility and related concepts: implications for clinical and forensic practice with deaf people. In S Austen and S Crocker (eds), *Deafness in Mind*, London, Whurr.

O'Rourke S, Gahir M, Reed R, Monteiro B *et al.* (2005) *Prison Scoping Exercise*. Unpublished report for the Department of Health.

O'Rourke S, Grewer F (2005) Assessment of deaf people in forensic mental health settings: a risky business. *The Journal of Forensic Psychiatry and Psychology* 16(4): 671–84.

Trafford Today (December 2005) *Police Meet with Deaf Residents*, issue 63, Trafford Metropolitan Borough Council, http://www.trafford.gov.uk/news/ issues/63/articles/police_meet_deaf_residents.asp, accessed 21 April 2006.

Vernon M and Miller K (2005) Obstacles faced by deaf people in the criminal justice system. *American Annals of the Deaf* 150(3): 283–91.

Vernon M, Steinberg AG, Montoya LA (2000) Deaf murderers: clinical and forensic issues. *Behavioural Sciences and the Law* 17(4): 495–516.

Wechsler D (1997) *Wechsler Adult Intelligence Scale* (3rd edn.), Oxford, Harcourt Assessment.

Winter BL (1980) Should deaf, blind serve as jurors? *Lawscope* 66: 133–4.

Young A, Howarth P, Ridgeway S, Monteiro B (2001) Forensic Referrals to the three specialist psychiatric units for deaf people in the UK. *Journal of Forensic Psychiatry*.

Young A, Monteiro B, Ridgeway S (2000) Deaf people with mental health needs in the criminal justice system: a review of the UK literature. *Journal of Forensic Psychiatry* 11(3): 556–70.

17

High Secure Care for Deaf People in England and Wales

MANJIT GAHIR

INTRODUCTION

This chapter will outline the provision of psychiatric services, especially high secure services, in England and Wales across the ages, with specific attention paid to those services for Deaf people. Consideration is given to the relationship between violence, mental illness and deafness, and whether equivalent numbers of Deaf to hearing people are housed in prisons or high secure psychiatric units. It will be argued that, in order to reduce aggressive incidents and respect the patients' human rights, services for Deaf people should be adapted to meet their unique communication and educational needs. It will be concluded that this is best achieved through specialist rather than integrated wards. A glossary is included at the end of the chapter.

PROVISION OF PSYCHIATRIC SERVICES IN ENGLAND AND WALES

The provision of psychiatric care in England and Wales has been changing since the 1960s with the closure of the large Victorian asylums and a move towards the integration of services within general medical hospitals or the provision of small, open, community-based psychiatric units.

Deafness and Challenging Behaviour: The 360° Perspective. Edited by S. Austen and D. Jeffery
© 2007 John Wiley & Sons Ltd

ALTERNATIVES TO HIGH SECURE PSYCHIATRIC UNITS

For patients who are behaviourally disturbed or aggressive, most general psychiatric units will have more highly staffed, and sometimes locked, psychiatric intensive care units (PICUs). Since 1975, there has been an increase in the number of beds for offender patients in medium secure units (MSUs). These are stand-alone psychiatric hospitals, which have an increased level of perimeter security, usually by means of a single fence of at least 4.7 m height. This type of unit will generally admit patients from prisons, the courts or police stations and occasionally from the community. They will also sometimes transfer patients from other community-based psychiatric units or PICUs if their risks of violence or absconding are too high to be managed there. The length of stay in MSUs is on average two to three years and some, but not all, will continue to manage patients after discharge into the community. The National Health Service (NHS) currently provides approximately 1500 medium secure beds in the UK, with a further 270 provided by the private sector. There are no specialist NHS medium secure beds for Deaf people although there are 32 in the private sector.

HIGH SECURE UNITS

The Secretary of State for Health is required by law (NHS Act 1977) to provide special (high secure) hospitals for detained mentally disordered patients, who in his or her opinion require treatment under conditions of special security on account of their dangerous, violent or criminal propensities. In order to be admitted to a high secure hospital, a patient has to be suffering from a mental disorder (defined in the Mental Health Act 1983 (HMSO, 1983) as Mental Illness, Psychopathic Disorder, Mental Impairment or Severe Mental Impairment), to be liable to detention under the Mental Health Act 1983 and to be regarded as a grave and immediate danger to the general public if at large, and who cannot be managed within conditions of lesser security. The types of behaviour that would warrant detention in high security would include serious assaults on members of the public, serious sexual assaults, threats to kill others, arson, use of poisons, sadistic behaviour, use of weapons or firearms, hostage-taking or persistent absconding from other secure establishments. The majority of patients admitted to high security come from prisons and medium secure psychiatric units, with a smaller number coming from low secure or open units. At this time, patients are not admitted directly to high security from the community.

LEVELS OF OFFENDING AMONGST DEAF PEOPLE

The law should stand the same, whether it is for Deaf or hearing people. In theory, Deaf people should receive exactly the same justice and sentencing as hearing people. However, there is reason to think this may not be the case. In practice the law is written with hearing people in mind and does not take into account the effects of deafness, which can affect the Deaf person's life experiences, offending behaviour and treatment by the criminal justice services. Although there is some evidence that Deaf people are treated leniently by the police (Vernon and Greenberg, 1999), there is mounting evidence that they are overrepresented in secure psychiatric care both in the UK and the USA. In a maximum secure facility in the USA, Harry and Dietz (1985) found the prevalence of Deaf people to be 5.1 per 1000, which is five times higher than the general population. Young *et al.* (2000) report the rate in England and Wales to be 12.3 per 1000, or twelve times higher than the hearing population. Other studies have noted an overrepresentation of certain types of offences, for example Miller and Vernon (2003) report that approximately 42% of Deaf offenders in a maximum secure facility in the USA were convicted of a sexual offence. Young *et al.* (2001) found that 38.6% of Deaf people referred to psychiatric services between 1968 and 1998 had been convicted of a sexual offence, which is greater than that expected from the general population. In 2001/2002, 12% of patients admitted to secure psychiatric facilities had a conviction for, or were charged with, sexual offences (Howard and Christopherson, 2003).

TYPES OF MENTAL DISORDER

All patients in high security are detained under the Mental Health Act 1983 or occasionally the Criminal Procedure (Insanity and Unfitness to Plead) Act 1991 (HMSO, 1991) and in order to be detained in hospital need to fulfil a number of criteria.

1. They must be suffering from an identifiable mental disorder.
2. That disorder must be treatable and require treatment in hospital.
3. Detention is required for the patient's own health, their own safety or for the safety of other people.

The Mental Health Act 1983 subdivides mental disorder into four categories: Mental Illness, Psychopathic Disorder, Mental Impairment and Severe Mental Impairment. It must be noted that these are legal terms and definitions and are not always in clinical usage.

MENTAL ILLNESS

This is not defined in the Mental Health Act and is left as a matter for clinical judgement. Clearly, there are a number of diagnosable mental illnesses ranging from anxiety disorders and other neuroses through to severe psychotic illnesses such as schizophrenia or mania. Detention is most likely to occur with the most serious illnesses but can apply to the non-psychotic illnesses, as long as the other detention criteria are met.

PSYCHOPATHIC DISORDER

This is defined in the Act as 'a persistent disorder or disability of mind (whether or not including significant impairment of intelligence), which results in abnormally aggressive or seriously irresponsible conduct'. Psychopathic Disorder is generally taken to equate to personality disorders: most commonly dissocial personality disorders and borderline personality disorder, although other types of personality disorder may also be included within the classification of Psychopathic Disorder.

MENTAL IMPAIRMENT

This is defined as 'a state of arrested or incomplete development of mind (not amounting to Severe Mental Impairment), which includes significant impairment of intelligence and social functioning and is associated with abnormally aggressive or seriously irresponsible conduct'. This is generally taken to equate to mild to moderate learning disability, and it must be noted that the violent behaviour has to be severe to warrant detention in a high secure hospital, as described on p. 276 above.

SEVERE MENTAL IMPAIRMENT

This is defined as 'a state of arrested or incomplete development of mind, which includes severe impairment of intelligence and social functioning and is associated with abnormally aggressive or seriously irresponsible conduct'. This is taken to equate to moderate to severe learning disability, but patients who are this learning-disabled are unlikely to require treatment in high security.

Clearly, these definitions of mental disorder are written in legal rather than clinical language and a degree of interpretation is needed when applying the Mental Health Act to clinical situations.

MENTAL DISORDER AND DEAFNESS

Little is known about the prevalence of these respective disorders in Deaf people. It is thought that Deaf people have at least the same prevalence of mental health problems as hearing people (Kitson and Thacker, 2000) and are likely to have a higher prevalence of schizophrenia than hearing people (Gray and du Feu, 2004). Braden (1994) reports that a meta analysis of 324 reports of mean Intelligence Quotient (IQ) for hearing-impaired people gave a grand-mean IQ of 97.14, which is significantly lower than the mean of 100 for hearing subjects, but adds that in practical terms the significance of this difference is marginal. Other investigators (Brauer *et al.*, 1998) comment that IQ is hard to accurately assess in Deaf people for a number of reasons, including the psychologist's inability to communicate in the appropriate language, the effect on the test results of using sign language interpreters and the paucity of tests validated on Deaf people. Given that 40% of Deaf people have additional disabilities (Crocker and Edwards, 2004) and that many of the causes of deafness can also result in traumatic brain damage, this may mean that the prevalence of severe mental impairment is likely to be higher than in hearing people. Certainly, diagnosis of mental disorder in Deaf people is particularly difficult because the widely used nosological system, e.g. DSM-IV (American Psychiatric Association, 1994) and ICD-10 (World Health Organization, 1992) are culturally based and do not take account of differences in symptomatology or presentation in Deaf people (O'Rourke and Grewer, 2005). They also note that the diagnosis of personality disorder is vulnerable to cultural bias. As a result, they say 'Deaf' characteristics may be viewed either as indicative of personality disorder or, conversely, a particular deviant behaviour may be excused even when it is also considered deviant in the Deaf community.

Aside from their possible higher prevalence of mental disorder, Deaf people may be over represented in high secure psychiatric provision because of historical gaps in the criminal justice system. This would also seem likely as Deaf people charged with a serious offence are more likely than hearing people to be found unfit to plead (Young *et al.*, 2001). Until 1991, any person found unfit to plead was by law detained indefinitely in a high secure psychiatric hospital. Fortunately, that law was changed with the advent of the Criminal Procedure Act 1991 (HMSO, 1991), which has meant that detention in high security is no longer automatic.

THE RELATIONSHIP BETWEEN MENTAL DISORDER AND VIOLENCE

There are well-established links between the presence of mental disorder and interpersonal violence, as well as violence to self (Swanson *et al.*, 1990; Hodgins, 1992). The exact nature of these links is still the subject of debate as it is clear that certain illnesses or symptoms are more related to violence than others (Taylor *et al.*, 1998; Taylor and Gunn, 1999). The disorders most linked to violent offending include alcohol and substance misuse, antisocial personality disorder and schizophrenia. Within schizophrenia, delusions are most significantly linked to violence. Other mental illnesses such as depression or bipolar affective disorder play a relatively small part in interpersonal violence although both are linked to self-harm and suicide.

Annual statistics for mentally disordered offenders are collected by the Home Office. The statistics for 2002 (Howard and Christopherson, 2003) demonstrate that 985 patients were admitted to a secure hospital under some form of restriction order, of which 72% were diagnosed as suffering from mental illness and 14% from some form of psychopathic disorder. The types of offences that result in detention in hospital include interpersonal violence (24.6%), robbery (9.6%), sexual offences (7.2%), murder (6.4%), other homicide (3.1%), arson (6.7%) and criminal damage (7.5%). It should be noted that offences by mentally ill offenders in the community form a small proportion (approximately 10%) of all violent offences or homicides, and this also appears to be true within psychiatric in-patient populations (Grassi, 2001).

HISTORY OF HIGH SECURE CARE IN ENGLAND AND WALES

There are currently three high secure psychiatric hospitals covering all of England and Wales, namely Broadmoor Hospital in Berkshire, Rampton Hospital in Nottinghamshire and Ashworth Hospital on

Merseyside. They provide beds for approximately one thousand mentally disordered patients, whose dangerous behaviour necessitates
treatment in conditions of high security. Of these bed-places, ten are
currently occupied by profoundly Deaf, sign-language-using male
patients, all located at Rampton Hospital.

BROADMOOR HOSPITAL

Broadmoor Hospital was first conceived in 1856 due to the lack of
provision for those deemed to be criminally insane and opened in 1863.
All of the patients there were detained under Her Majesty's pleasure
due to insanity, and Broadmoor Hospital was the only high secure
psychiatric institution serving the whole of England and Wales. Between
1860 and 1910, the number of patients at Broadmoor Hospital increased
from 500 to 840, requiring the building of a second hospital in England.
Currently, Broadmoor Hospital has 395 beds and provides services to
men with mental illness, men with psychopathic disorder as well as
some women patients.

RAMPTON HOSPITAL

Rampton Hospital is located near the town of Retford in north
Nottinghamshire and was designed to relieve the overcrowding at
Broadmoor. It opened in 1912 and admitted a number of mentally ill
patients from Broadmoor Hospital. From 1920, it only admitted people
with learning disability, those convicted of an offence or those who
were not manageable in general learning-disability hospitals but who
were detained under provision of the Mental Deficiency Act 1913
(HMSO, 1913). In 1947, Rampton Hospital transferred to the Ministry
of Health under provision of the NHS Act 1946 (HMSO, 1946) but
the hospital continued to be managed by the Board of Control. At the
present time, Rampton Hospital has 382 beds and is divided into five
directorates including Mental Illness (which contains the Deaf unit),
the Learning Disability Services, Personality Disorder Service,
Dangerous and Severe Personality Disorder Unit (all of which are for
male patients), and the Womens' Service Directorate, which admits
approximately 50 female patients.

ASHWORTH HOSPITAL

What is now Ashworth Hospital was formed by the amalgamation in
1990 of two hospitals, namely Moss Side Hospital (built in 1914) and

Park Lane Hospital (built in 1987). Moss Side Hospital was initially opened with the intention of admitting those with learning disability or epilepsy, but during World War I over 3000 patients suffering from 'shell shock' were admitted and treated there. One hundred patients were transferred there from Rampton Hospital in 1933 due to over-crowding, and Moss Side continued to grow, such that by the end of World War II it housed 375 inpatients. Ashworth Hospital currently has 295 beds for men with mental illness and men with personality disorder.

HIGH SECURE DEAF UNIT, RAMPTON HOSPITAL

Regrettably, records have never been kept on how many profoundly Deaf patients have been admitted to each high secure psychiatric hos-pital. It can be assumed that since Rampton Hospital historically admitted patients with learning disabilities and other disabilities a number of Deaf patients would have been admitted. It is known that Deaf sign-language-using patients have been admitted to Rampton Hospital since the 1970s, all of whom suffered from mental disorder and had either committed serious offences such as rape, homicide, arson or sexual abuse or were not able to be managed in other units due to severe aggression. Rampton employed its first Deaf support worker in 1983 in the Education Department. Over the years, an exper-tise in the assessment and treatment of Deaf offenders has developed in Rampton Hospital with the employment of sign language interpret-ers, Deaf support workers and a Deaf development worker, who are involved with experienced hearing staff in outside assessments and in-patient therapy.

Following the publication of the findings of the Daniel Joseph Inquiry (Mishcon *et al.*, 2000) into the killing of an elderly woman by a young profoundly Deaf man in London, the Government responded with the publication of the consultation document *A Sign of the Times* (Department of Health, 2002). In this document Rampton Hospital is identified as being the sole national provider of high secure psychiatric services for prelingually Deaf sign language users. This position was reiterated in the finalised document *Mental Health and Deafness: Towards Equity and Access* (Department of Health, 2005), and since 2004 Deaf patients requiring high secure care have only been admitted to Rampton Hospital. Initially, the Deaf patients in Rampton were on different wards depending on their Mental Health Act classification.

However, they were then all moved to the Mental Health Directorate (male mental illness) due to the number of recurrent problems being identified. These included patients' isolation and frustration, lack of staff specialisation and variable access to education and other therapies. In September 2002, all of the Deaf patients moved together to the High Secure Deaf Unit, which was set up on a therapeutic community model, using British Sign Language as the language of choice. The therapeutic community model has been used in prisons (Woodward, 1999) and other secure units in the Netherlands and the USA with some success (Dolan and Coid, 1993). It was chosen to try to empower a generally disempowered and disadvantaged group of patients by means of democracy, a flattened hierarchy, a spirit of enquiry and permissiveness and reality confrontation. Fundamental to this is a respect for cultural diversity and the availability of communication support for Deaf staff and patients.

As with hearing patients, Deaf patients within high security services will suffer from one of, or a combination of, mental disorders that may increase their potential for violence. Miller and Vernon (2003) speculate on a number of factors that might lead to violence amongst Deaf people including young age at incarceration, constricted vocabulary, limited education, anger towards themselves and society in general, brain damage and learning disabilities. Within high secure Deaf services these factors are also relevant but there are two factors above any that appear to be most relevant in precipitating violence in Deaf patients.

These are:

- communication frustration
- educational limitations.

COMMUNICATION FRUSTRATION

Taylor (2001) suggests that violence may be used as a language substitute in the general population as well as in those with mental disorder, and she regards the fact of men being more violent than women as possibly due to earlier language development in girls compared to boys. Also noted is the higher incidence of violence in certain disorders where concurrent expressive language disorders are prevalent, such as autism and schizophrenia. Furthermore, people with disruption of interpersonal communication are less likely to have a social network and more likely to manifest interpersonal violence. Frustration at not being able to communicate one's needs or wants can lead to aggression and is highlighted by the case example below.

Case Study: Mr A

Mr A is a 41-year-old man who was sentenced to three years' imprisonment for assault and making threats to kill. During the course of that sentence, he was made subject to further charges of assault and making threats to rape and was ultimately admitted to the High Secure Deaf Unit and detained on a Hospital Order. During the course of two years in prison, Mr A perpetrated approximately 500 assaults or acts of violence on prison staff, as well as writing numerous notes threatening to kill them or rape the female staff. While in prison, he did not have any Deaf visitors or input from a sign language interpreter. All communication with him was either by pointing and miming or by writing notes. Mr A spent almost two years in segregation in prison and was not allowed contact with other prisoners. Conversely, in the High Secure Deaf Unit, he very quickly integrated with the other Deaf patients and had only two very brief periods of seclusion following assaults on staff early on in his admission. He communicates fluently and effectively in BSL and is able to control his anger by engaging in one-to-one therapy and group work. The major factor that Mr A identifies as the cause of his assaultive behaviour in prison is the fact that no one could communicate effectively with him and he had no other way of making his wishes and frustrations known.

The key to preventing or diffusing violent incidents is communication, and in this regard the use of Deaf support staff, relay interpreters and sign language interpreters is extremely important. Only through the establishment of the High Secure Deaf Unit have we been able to focus on the language-dependent intricacies of aggression prevention. A number of factors might suggest that a patient is becoming angry or disturbed. These include forceful, angry signing, loud vocalisation, finger pointing, staring, invading personal space, striking or banging objects and using offensive or threatening language. A sophisticated knowledge of sign language is crucial to spot these triggers in a Deaf person. It is imperative that once these signs are recognised the patient should be asked what is bothering them and what can be done to help.

If the patient is to feel 'heard', staff must be fluent in sign language or be skilled in using sign language interpreters. Similarly, the sign language interpreters will need specialist skill and experience in working with this client group. An important forum where problems can be identified and dealt with early on is the daily community meeting, which involves all of the patients on the ward, the staff and sign language interpreters. The meeting is chaired by one of the patients and allows a protected environment where problems such as bullying or use of abusive language can be discussed and resolved.

Communication not only benefits the Deaf patient by reducing their frustration but also allows the staff to get to know the patient better, and in doing so prepare strategies for reducing or preventing violence. One of the most important factors in reducing the likelihood of violence or disturbed behaviour is having an in-depth knowledge of the patients: their current state and their history. Linguistic and educational limitations may mean that the patient is not a good historian. However, if the Deaf patient has been away to boarding school it may also mean that their families are not able to fill in the gaps in the historical information. Most schools destroy their records of students after only a few years, thus a full history may be difficult to take. Native Deaf signers are likely to be more successful in eliciting this information than hearing staff or interpreters.

Regrettably, there are times when, despite all efforts at communication, prevention and de-escalation, a violent incident may take place. At times of extreme violence, and in a last resort, the patient in the High Secure Deaf Unit would be restrained using a five-person team. The use of control and restraint is managed via hospital policies and all staff who are involved must attend a five-day training course with annual refresher courses. Additional courses in managing people who are using weapons and the use of protective equipment and shields are also available. This training is available to all members of Deaf staff as well as hearing staff, although not to sign language interpreters, who have a different role to play as communication facilitators when patients are restrained.

Following a violent incident, the outcome may be that the underlying cause of the violence is resolved and the patient returns to the main ward environment. However, in the case of ongoing threats of violence or disturbed behaviour, the patient may be secluded in a purpose-built, locked room, expressly to prevent others from significant harm. Seclusion is not a treatment and is never used as punishment or retribution or solely in response to self-harm. It is used only as a last resort, when all other alternative approaches have been exhausted and takes place for the shortest time period possible. One of the difficulties encountered in the Deaf service in relation to seclusion is the ongoing communication with patients. The seclusion room may utilise low-level lighting to aid relaxation but this can make communicating in sign language very difficult. The fact that patients and staff are communicating via a small window in a locked door can impair the quality of information communicated and the relationship between staff and patients, and it is therefore essential that normal, open communication be resumed as quickly as possible. The use of seclusion is monitored internally by the hospital and externally by the Mental Health Act Commission, and it is notable that the rate of seclusion in the Deaf Unit is extremely low. The reasons for this are still speculative, but might be related to the Deaf Unit having a relatively stable long-term population when compared to the admission wards in Rampton Hospital, to the skills of staff who know the patients well and who are able to de-escalate a potentially violent situation early on but perhaps, most importantly, to the communication that is facilitated by interpreters and Deaf support staff.

EDUCATION AND GROUP WORK

Deaf people often suffer from educational impairment despite input from specialist Deaf schools. Lack of a formal education may be compounded by a lack of incidental learning and may result in an inability to 'verbalise' internal feelings, resentment and anger towards peers and regarding those in authority as 'not listening'. It is notable that within the High Secure Deaf Service, none of the Deaf patients holds any sort of formal qualification and, although the majority attended residential Deaf schools, most are barely literate in English. There is a very strong education department in Rampton Hospital that uses hearing staff to teach Deaf patients various subjects including basic literacy and numeracy, cookery, life skills and sex education. All of the sessions are aided by an interpreter and Deaf support worker, with the notable exception of computing skills, which are taught by a Deaf member of staff. Prior to September 2003 and setting up of the High Secure Deaf Unit, patients were able to access education but this was fragmented and took place in a separate education department. The majority of lessons now take place on the Deaf Unit; this allows increased interaction between patients, staff and teachers. The learning can be reinforced by peers and is thus more Deaf-orientated and realistic.

There is also an increased access to group work that is specific to their developmental needs, such as a world news and media group, emotions and coping with anger group and a healthy lifestyles group looking at ways to stop smoking and lose weight. Work is currently ongoing to adapt various programmes used to treat different offending behaviours such as a sex offender treatment programme, arson group and violent offender treatment programme. Until these group work programmes are fully operational, patients continue to engage in one-to-one therapy with psychologists and nursing staff.

CONCLUSION

Deaf people may have an increased prevalence of mental disorder, which is disproportionately associated with violence. Owing to discrimination within the 'fitness to plead' legislation prior to 1991, people who were deemed unfit to plead were automatically incarcerated in high secure services rather than being given prison sentences or being released. This resulted in an overrepresentation of Deaf people in high security hospitals.

The development of the High Secure Deaf Unit within Rampton Hospital represents a turning point in the history of high secure services for Deaf people nationally and exemplifies recognition of the fundamental rights of the Deaf patient. The recognition of the linguistic and educational limitations and needs of this client group has resulted in vast improvements in service provision and in a low incidence of violent incidents on the Deaf Unit when compared to prisons or other units within Rampton Hospital.

REFERENCES

American Psychiatric Association (1994) *Diagnostic and Statistical Manual of Mental Disorders*, Washington, American Psychiatric Association.
Braden JP (1994) *Deafness, Deprivation and IQ*, New York, Plenum Press.
Brauer A, Braden JP, Pollard RQ, Hardy-Braz ST (1998) Deaf and hard of hearing people. In Sandoval J, Frisby CL, Geisinger KF, Scheuneman JD, Grenier JR (eds), *Test Interpretation and Diversity: Achieving Equity in Assessment*, Washington, American Psychological Association, pp. 297–315.
Crocker S, Edwards L (2004) Deafness and additional difficulties. In Austen S, Crocker S (eds), *Deafness in Mind: Working Psychologically with Deaf People Across the Lifespan*, London, Whurr, pp. 252–69.

Department of Health (2002) *A Sign of the Times: Modernising Mental Health Services for People who are Deaf*, London, Department of Health.

Department of Health (2004) National Health Service Act 1977: Primary Care Trust Medical Services (No. 2): Directions 2004, http://www.dh.gov. uk/PublicationsAndStatistics/Publications/PublicationsLegislation/Public ationsLegislationArticle/fs/en?CONTENT ID=4094212&chk=qcCqJO, accessed 30 June 2006.

Department of Health (2005) *Mental Health and Deafness, Towards Equity and Access*, London, Department of Health.

Dolan B, Coid J (1993) *Psychopathy and Antisocial Personality Disorders: Treatment and Research Issues*, London, Gaskell.

Grassi L (2001) Characteristics of violent behaviour in acute psychiatric in-patients: a 5-year Italian study. *Acta Psychiatrica Scandinavica* 104(4): 273–9.

Gray A, du Feu M (2004) The causes of schizophrenia and its implications for deaf people. In Austen S, Crocker S (eds), *Deafness in Mind. Working Psychologically with Deaf People Across the Lifespan*, London, Whurr, pp. 206–21.

Harry B, Dietz PE (1985) Offenders in a silent world: hearing impairment and deafness in relation to criminality, incompetence and insanity. *Bulletin for the American Academy of Psychiatry and the Law* 13(1): 85–162.

HMSO (1913) *The Mental Deficiency Act 1913*, London, HMSO.

HMSO (1946) *The National Health Service Act 1946*, London, HMSO.

HMSO (1983) *The Mental Health Act 1983*, London, TSO.

HMSO (1991) Criminal Procedure (Insanity and Unfitness to Plead) Act (1991) http://www.opsi.gov.uk/ACTS/acts 1991/UKpga_19910025_en_1. htm, accessed 26 June 2006.

Hodgins S (1992) Mental disorder, intellectual deficiency and crime. Evidence from a birth cohort. *Archives of General Psychiatry* 49(6): 476–83.

Howard D, Christopherson O (2003) *Statistics of Mentally Disordered Offenders 2002: England and Wales*, London, Home Office.

Kitson N, Thacker A (2000) Adult Psychiatry. In Hindley P, Kitson N (eds), *Mental Health and Deafness*, London, Whurr, pp. 75–98.

Miller K, Vernon M (2003) Deaf offenders in a prison population. *Journal of Deaf Studies and Deaf Education* 8(3): 357–62.

Mishcon J, Sensky T, Lindsey M, Cook S (2000) *Report of the Independent Inquiry Team into the Care and Treatment of Daniel Joseph*, London, Merton Sutton and Wandsworth Health Authority.

O'Rourke S, Grewer G (2005) Assessment of deaf people in forensic mental health settings: a risky business! *Journal of Forensic Psychiatry and Psychology* 16(4): 671–84.

Swanson JW, Holzer CF, Ganju VK (1990) Violence and psychiatric disorder in the community: evidence from the Epidemiologic Catchment Area surveys. *Hospital and Community Psychiatry* 41(7): 761–70.

Taylor PJ (2001) Human communication, language and mental illness. In France J, Kramer S (eds), *Communication and Mental Illness: Theoretical and Practical Approaches*, London, Jessica Kingsley, pp. 325–34.

Taylor PJ, Gunn J (1999) Homicides by people with mental illness: myth and reality. *British Journal of Psychiatry* 174: 9–14.

Taylor PJ, Lees M, Williams D, Butterwell M *et al.* (1998) Mental disorder and violence: a special (high security) hospital study. *British Journal of Psychiatry* 172: 218–26.

Vernon M, Greenberg SF (1999) Violence in deaf and hard of hearing people: a review of the literature. *Aggression and Violent Behaviour* 4(3): 259–72.

Woodward R (1999) The prison communities: therapy within a custodial setting. In Campling P, Haigh R (eds), *Therapeutic Communities Past, Present and Future*, London, Jessica Kingsley, pp. 151–62.

World Health Organization (1992) *The ICD-10 Classification of Mental and Behavioural Disorders: Clinical Descriptions and Diagnostic Guidelines*, Geneva, World Health Organization.

Young A, Howarth P, Ridgeway S, Monteiro B (2001) Forensic referrals to the three specialist psychiatric units for deaf people in the UK. *Journal of Forensic Psychiatry* 12(1): 19–35.

Young A, Monteiro B, Ridgeway S (2000) Deaf people with mental health needs in the criminal justice system: a review of the UK literature. *Journal of Forensic Psychiatry* 11(3): 556–70.

GLOSSARY

Board of Control – a Government department introduced in 1913 with national responsibility for provision of psychiatric services in England and Wales. In 1948, its responsibilities passed to the Ministry for Health **apart** from for the management of the three high secure hospitals. These moved to the Ministry for Health upon the dissolution of the Board of Control in 1960.

Criminal Procedure (Insanity and Unfitness to Plead) Act 1991 – An Act of Parliament for England and Wales that makes provision for persons who are unfit to be tried in court or who are found 'not guilty' of an offence by virtue of insanity. Since April 2005, the case is heard by a senior judge sitting alone, who is required to hear expert psychiatric evidence on the presence or absence of mental disorder, hears a trial of the facts of a case and will decide on disposal. There is discretion in disposal, which ranges from an acquittal, through community or probation orders, to compulsory admission to a secure psychiatric hospital.

Home Office – a department of the British Government that deals with internal affairs in England and Wales including law and order, immigration and provision for mentally disordered offenders. There is a specific department within the Home Office called the Mental Health Unit that deals with the transfer of prisoners to secure psychiatric hospitals and the powers of the Home Secretary under sections 41 of the Mental Health Act 1983 (see below).

Hospital Order – this is a sentence passed by a court on a person who is found to be mentally disordered at the time of sentencing under provision of section 37 of the Mental Health Act 1983. The judge must be satisfied, on the evidence of two registered medical practitioners, one of whom must have special knowledge in the treatment of psychiatric disorders, that the defendant is suffering from a mental disorder, which is of a nature or degree that makes it appropriate for her or him to be detained in hospital for medical treatment and that a hospital order is the most suitable method of dealing with the case. In cases where the judge feels that the defendant poses a serious risk of harm to the public, a restriction order may be added to the hospital order under section 41 of the Act.

Learning Disability – also called mental retardation. A condition of arrested or incomplete development of mind including impairment of skills in cognitive, motor, language and social fields.

Mental Deficiency Act 1913 – Legislation for England and Wales that defined the types of 'mental defectives' and made provision for their detention in institutions. Also established the Board of Control (see above).

Mental Health Act 1983 – Legislation for England and Wales that allows the compulsory detention of people suffering from mental disorder, and puts into place statutory safeguards for review of their detention and their compulsory treatment with medication.

Mental Health Act Commission – Statutory body that has responsibility for reviewing the implementation of the Mental Health Act 1983 in relation to detained patients in England and Wales.

National Health Service (NHS) – The NHS began in 1948 by Act of Parliament. Most hospitals in the UK had previously been operated as non-profit-making concerns. With the NHS Act, these were all compulsorily acquired and subsequently administered by the State, and all treatments became universally available at no cost at the point of provision, the whole being centrally funded by taxation. From 1948 on, all hospital doctors, hospital nurses and all other hospital staff became salaried employees of the State.

Restriction Orders – this is an order that can be added to a hospital order in cases where there is a need to protect the public from serious harm, and it can last for a specified time period or can be without limit of time in serious cases. The patient may not be given leave of absence from the hospital without the Home Secretary's consent and cannot be discharged from hospital unless authorised by the Home Secretary or a mental health review tribunal.

Secretary of State for Health – British Government minister with overall responsibility for health policy in the UK.

18

Risk Assessment and Risk Management with Deaf People

SUE O'ROURKE

INTRODUCTION

The focus of risk research has, in recent years, shifted from the pursuit of accurate risk prediction towards risk management. The goal is to develop tools that enable clinicians to manage risk effectively. Research into mental health and deafness is generally sparse; the field of risk and deafness is no exception.

This chapter outlines risk assessment and risk management, as it relates to hearing offenders, and reasons are given for doubting the applicability of some of this research to deaf people. Caution is needed when applying 'best practice' in risk management from hearing research; deaf-specific factors need to be built into the consideration of risk.

In this instance 'deaf' refers to those people who were born deaf or deafened at an early age, before the development of speech, many of whom see themselves as part of a cultural and linguistic minority, using sign language and being members of the Deaf community. 'Risk' in this context is risk of harm to others. The issues of self-harm and suicide are not dealt with in this chapter.

Deafness and Challenging Behaviour: The 360° Perspective. Edited by S. Austen and D. Jeffery
© 2007 John Wiley & Sons Ltd

WHAT ARE 'RISK MANAGEMENT' AND 'RISK ASSESSMENT'?

WHY MANAGE RISK?

At any point in time there are numerous individuals detained in hospitals under the compulsory powers of the Mental Health Act 1983 (Department of Health and Welsh Office, 1999) due to the judgement that they are likely to be at risk of harming others. Assessments made by professionals about who is likely to be violent have huge implications for the person whose liberty is under threat, and for society as a whole, containing as it does potential victims.

The political climate of the day has an impact on risk assessment. If risk prediction were 95% accurate, for every 100 people detained, five would not present a risk and so be detained needlessly. There is no public outcry or tabloid outrage about such instances. However, if five out of 100 people who are released into the community re-offend violently, this has devastating effects on the victims and is considered an unacceptable error rate. We are therefore called upon to develop more accurate measures of risk and more robust procedures for its management.

CLINICAL JUDGEMENT

Clinicians make judgements about risk on a daily basis: should I visit this person at home? Can I be alone with this person in a room on the ward? Am I the best person to deliver bad news to this person? Generally, clinicians feel very comfortable with their own abilities to make these judgements. However, research in the area of risk has shown that clinical judgement alone is a poor predictor of whether a previously violent individual continues to present a risk to others (Gardner *et al.*, 1996). One possible reason is that clinicians tend to focus on current presentation rather than taking a longitudinal view. The patient who is stable and well behaved on the ward, who has not offended while detained, may seem a safe bet. However, behaviour occurs in specific contexts; institutional life can be safe, secure, structured and predictable. Life on the outside is very different. Exposure to destabilisers such as alcohol, drugs, relationships, access to victims and family pressures can replicate the conditions around previous offending and can move the individual closer to re-offending.

The therapeutic relationship with the individual can also affect clinical judgement relating to risk. This may be particularly relevant in cases of psychopathic personality disorder where the presentation is characterised by superficial charm, conning and manipulative behaviour and pathological lying. In such cases, risk judgements are more accurate when carried out by a clinician not involved in the treatment of the patient (Hare, 1991).

ACTUARIAL RISK ASSESSMENT

Actuarial risk assessment was developed in response to findings that clinical judgement is a poor predictor of risk.

Based on studies of re-offending rates, research such as the Oakridge study (Harris *et al.*, 1993) has shown that the presence of certain factors in the individual's background contribute to an increased risk of recidivism. These historical or 'static' risk factors include those relating to the individual's early life, mental health diagnoses, previous offending and behaviour and previous responses to intervention and supervision.

Various psychometric tools have been developed based solely on static risk factors, for example the Violence Risk Appraisal Guide (VRAG) (Harris *et al.*, 1993) or the Static-99 (Hanson and Thornton, 1999). These tools provide a percentage probability that someone will re-offend within a given time, based on research on groups of offenders previously released. Proponents would argue that this is all that is required in the measurement of risk. However, the usefulness of these measures is limited. From a clinical point of view such tools are unsatisfactory, since the individual is damned for ever by virtue of their history, with no possibility of change. Common sense dictates that risk occurs in a context, whereas these measures take no account of this and therefore have little to say about risk management.

STRUCTURED CLINICAL JUDGEMENT

Third-generation risk assessment acknowledges the importance of research evidence in relation to actuarial risk prediction, but combines this with a consideration of clinical presentation and the environment in which the violence may occur. Thus, we move from risk prediction and assessment to risk management.

In terms of assessing risk of physical violence in individuals with a previous violent offence, the HCR-20 (Webster *et al.*, 1997) offers a means of structured clinical judgement. This tool combines historical/ static risk factors known to be associated with violent recidivism (H) with relevant aspects of current clinical presentation, or dynamic factors (C). The risk is considered in relation to specific environment and risk-management items (R) and may relate to risk inside an institution or in the community. Obviously, historical items remain the same over time. Clinical items may change with intervention, as may risk-management items. It is recommended that the HCR-20 is re-evaluated every six months or when a change in location is being considered, whichever is the sooner. Interrater reliability is maximised by ensuring that raters have specific training and adhere to definitions in the manual. Items are rated on a scale from 0 to 2. The 20-item list is given in Table 18.1.

The aim of the HCR-20 is that not only does it enable the assessment of risk but it also points towards what is necessary in terms of risk management. A more recent tool, which takes this a step further, is the Risk of Sexual Violence Protocol (RSVP) developed by Hart *et al.* (2003). This looks at static factors related to sexually violent recidivism in convicted sex offenders, combined with clinical presentation. However, the risk-management process is enhanced by the inclusion of possible imagined futures in which risk may occur. Used within a multidisciplinary team, this can enable a consideration of risk scenarios and the development of strategies for effective management.

Table 18.1   HCR-20 items

Historical items	Clinical items	Risk-management items
Previous violence	Lack of insight	Plans lack feasibility
Young age at first violent incident	Negative attitudes	Exposure to destabilisers
Relationship instability	Active symptoms of major mental illness	Lack of personal support
Employment problems		Non-compliance with remediation attempts
Substance misuse problems	Impulsivity	Stress
Major mental illness	Unresponsive to treatment	
Psychopathy		
Early maladjustment		
Personality disorder		
Prior supervision failure		

DEAF PEOPLE AND RISK

Are deaf people more likely to be violent than hearing people? There are no data with which to answer this question. Theoretically, the likelihood of being violent may be increased for a number of reasons. First of all, some causes of deafness may lead to increased risk: meningitis, rubella and anoxia at birth may all lead to additional brain damage, which may impact on self-regulatory mechanisms. Secondly, it could be argued that, owing to communication problems, deaf people have an inherently more stressful life, particularly in the area of interpersonal relationships. Therefore recourse to aggressive behaviour may be more likely. Thirdly, deaf people in a hearing environment lack access to learning in many instances. Research has shown that hearing parents of deaf children are more didactic and less discursive with them than with their hearing children (Gregory, 1978). Deaf people may arrive at adulthood with less of an understanding of social and emotional aspects of life and fewer coping strategies. This is not due to an inherent deficit but to a deprivation of opportunity. This view would be supported by the finding that the prevalence of behavioural difficulties is greater in deaf than in hearing children (Hindley, 1997).

The picture in relation to deaf adults is less clear, and whether these children later go on to offend is unknown. We know that, historically, deaf people have been over represented in high secure hospitals (Monteiro, 1999, personal communication) but this may be due to a lack of services at medium and low secure levels. Forensic referrals for deaf people have increased in recent years and continue to do so (Young *et al.*, 2001). However, this may in part be due to new services opening, which tend to identify previously unmet need and generate referrals.

Statistics relating to the number of deaf people going through the courts or in prison are not kept. A recent scoping exercise for the Department of Health (O'Rourke *et al.*, 2005a) suggests that, at the end of 2005, out of a prison population of approximately 76 000 there may be approximately 130 deaf prisoners. However, there are considerable difficulties in identifying deaf people in the prison system, and so this may be a gross underestimation. In addition, the scoping exercise was not able to distinguish deaf sign language users from deafened or hard-of-hearing prisoners. How many of these prisoners have committed a violent crime is not known.

One fairly robust finding is that, of the identified population of deaf people who have offended, there is an overrepresentation of sex offenders, particularly against minors (Young *et al.*, 2000). There are a number of suggestions in the literature about why this might be the case. These include the presence of aetiologies of deafness that can be associated with frontal lobe damage and hence an increased tendency towards impulsivity (Vernon and Rich, 1997). It has been suggested that the high incidence of sexual abuse perpetrated against deaf children is relevant here in so far as deaf children who have been abused or been exposed to abusive situations may not have had the opportunity to learn what is normal and abnormal, appropriate or inappropriate, in relationships, and thus grow up to become offenders against children themselves.

UNDERSTANDING DEAF FACTORS IN ASSESSING AND MANAGING RISK

In considering the risk posed by a deaf person with a prior history of violent or sexually violent offending, it is necessary to have an understanding of factors specific to deafness that may impact on risk. These may relate to the person themselves or to the environment in which the deaf person finds themselves, which, of course, includes other people. The factors considered below are theoretically relevant to risk, but as yet this is unproven.

FACTORS RELATING TO THE PERSON

Cause of Deafness

In people with impulsive aggression, a neuropsychology assessment is useful in identifying possible cognitive correlates that would support an organic component to the presentation. This would then have implications for management, assisting staff in developing realistic treatment goals and considering which aspects of the person's behaviour will require long-term management by external strategies.

Communication

Communication can impact on risk in a number of ways. An individual with minimal language skills needs to be assessed to ascertain whether this is due to learning disability, specific language disorder or a result of a history of deprivation. The result of this assessment helps to develop realistic treatment goals. For example, an individual with minimal language skills may not have the receptive language to under-stand the consequences of their behaviour or to engage in work related to building empathy.

Attitudes to Hearing People

Past frustrations or even abuse may lead the individual to have a very negative and hostile view of hearing people, sometimes mistaken for paranoia. This may lead to a general dislike of hearing people, suggest-ing that any hearing person who displays a discriminatory view or misunderstands deafness may be at risk. Alternatively, there may be specific plans to harm a named individual.

Deaf Cognitive Distortions

Offenders in general are often cognitively distorted, displaying atti-tudes and patterns of thinking that permit or excuse their offending. For example, a rapist may tell himself that most women secretly desire to be raped; an armed robber may assert that robbery is a 'victimless' crime as the bank or shop is insured. Deaf offenders may develop cognitive distortions relating to their deafness. For example, attitudes of entitlement may excuse behaviour, the deaf person telling them-selves that hearing people think they are stupid so deserve to suffer. A common distortion is that of blaming deafness for the behaviour, excus-ing offending by being deaf and 'not knowing any better'. This may be a highly successful strategy with which hearing professionals will collude. For example, a deaf man in his fifties was arrested after his daughter disclosed that he had been subjecting her to sexual abuse over many years. He told his solicitor that, as a deaf person, he had no way of explaining the 'facts of life' to his hearing daughter, and so was showing her instead. A specialist psychological assessment exposed this as a means of trying to use his deafness to excuse his behaviour.

Lack of Experience/Understanding

There are instances where issues of deprivation of knowledge and lack of understanding are relevant to an understanding of risk. Much of what hearing people learn is picked up incidentally by overhearing. The deaf person is disadvantaged by not being able to pick up informa-tion in this way and so may arrive at adulthood with striking gaps in knowledge and skills. Taking account of this is vital in planning risk management, in setting realistic and achievable targets, in not assuming the client has background knowledge and in planning services that meet the person's need.

FACTORS RELATING TO THE ENVIRONMENT

The Deaf Community

The Deaf community can undoubtedly provide support to the individual, and there are a number of projects around the country run by deaf people for deaf people that do this. However, fitting into a small community can be stressful. It is very difficult to be anonymous within such a small group of people, and for many individuals their offending is well known in Deaf circles making reintegration problematic at times. A particular area of concern is that, given the mix of age and gender found in the local Deaf club, this could be a means of accessing future victims for sex offenders against children, with social events giving ample opportunity for grooming.

A Hearing Environment

If the deaf individual is living in a hearing environment, this is inherently stressful, which is likely to increase risk. An additional complication is, while the individual's risk is gradually increasing, those around them are not able to communicate and therefore cannot adequately assess risk. This can have disastrous consequences. If it is unavoidable that a deaf offender be detained in a hearing environment, the risk-management plan must identify a package of support, which would minimise risk and increase the staff's ability to assess on an ongoing basis. This would include Deaf awareness training as a requirement for all staff (and offered to hearing patients), BSL training, the employment of deaf staff and access to interpreters.

Availability of Specialist Services

How easily the person can access specialist Deaf services may be relevant to the management of risk. Although social workers for deaf people may be available in the local area and do sterling work in supporting deaf people in the community, they rarely have mental health training or knowledge of forensic issues. Ongoing access to specialists in forensic mental health and deafness for both the individual and local practitioners is likely to improve the monitoring of risk.

DEAF PEOPLE AND RISK MEASURES

ISSUES OF VALIDITY

In considering using psychometric tools with deaf people, it is important to be aware that the validity of static factors in predicting risk has not yet been demonstrated. There are theoretical reasons why some historical items, strongly associated with recidivism in hearing offenders, may not demonstrate such an association in deaf people. Some examples are outlined below in relation to specific measures.

A second area of concern, in relation to validity, is that none of the measures, as they exist, take account of the deafness-specific factors as outlined above. Obviously, for a deaf person, their deafness, and all that is associated with it, is central to their personality and how they experience the world. Research is currently underway by the author to ascertain which, if any, of the deafness factors discussed are associated with violent re-offending. If any of these factors are associated with re-offending, specific risk measures will be developed to take account of this.

ISSUES OF RELIABILITY

Psychometric instruments, such as questionnaires, which rely on administering specific questions in a standardised manner, are extremely unreliable. Frequently, items cannot be translated simply into BSL without additional explanation. Although this is necessary in order that the person understands the question, in doing this the questionnaire is changed to such a degree that it can no longer be seen as standardised. In addition, the questionnaires having been developed with hearing people are not necessarily addressing issues relevant to deafness (O'Rourke and Grewer, 2005). It is recommended that this exercise in questionnaire translation with an individual deaf person should not even be attempted.

It is self-evident that the risk assessment is only as good as the information upon which it is based. Deaf people without access to specialist services may receive numerous erroneous diagnoses over time, which are then kept on file and become part of their clinical record. Measures that collate details of static risk factors then pick up these misdiagnoses which then become part of the risk assessment. In this way, previous errors and misjudgements can lead to current unreliable risk assessment.

SPECIFIC MEASURES

Psychometric tools used in a forensic setting often require specific training to be undertaken by the practitioner. Some of the most widely used tools are described below and their applicability to deaf people considered. Although this is by no means an exhaustive list, the issues in relation to deafness could be extrapolated to other measures.

HCR-20/SVR-20

These are 20-item instruments that combine historical or static risk factors with clinical presentation and a consideration of the risk environment. The HCR-20 (Webster *et al.*, 1997) deals with the risk of physical violence while the SVR-20 (Boer *et al.*, 1997) enables structured clinical judgement in relation to the risk of sexual violence.

There are no practical reasons why these two measures cannot be carried out on deaf people. However, as stated above, the validity of using tools based on research with hearing offenders is questionable. In rating the historical items, special attention needs to be paid to the quality of information obtained, for example by non-specialists.

Historical Items

When assessing deaf individuals, the meaningfulness of certain items has to be considered. For example, 'early maladjustment', predictive of re-offending, may have less potency among a deaf population, since difficulties in childhood are so prevalent (often due to the child being in a non-communicating environment, either at home or at school). Lack of communication and poor educational provision frequently lead to frustration and thus a higher incidence of being labelled as 'maladjusted', which may then be less predictive of who will or won't go on to offend or have problems later.

Similarly, problems in employment, which may have predictive power in a hearing population, may be less relevant in a deaf population, where underachievement may well reflect the lack of Deaf awareness in the environment and by employers, rather than the difficulties being located in the person themselves.

Clinical Items

When considering clinical items based on how the person presents 'lack of insight' or 'negative attitudes' can be rated as present, when in fact the difficulty is lack of knowledge or experience. Deaf culture is relevant here too. Deaf people can appear blunt compared with hearing (English) culture. This apparent bluntness can be interpreted as rudeness and, in terms of assessment, as displaying negative attitudes.

Non-compliance with treatment is rated under clinical items. It is important to note whether the treatment being offered is accessible and appropriate for a deaf person. A BSL user refusing to join a hearing anger management group could be considered non-compliant or just sensible!

Risk-management Items

The risk-management items of the HCR-20 and SVR-20 allow the clinician to take account of factors within the environment, which will affect risk. Being explicit about destabilising influences and stressors enables consideration about whether plans are feasible in terms of risk and a risk-management plan to be developed. With regard to deaf people, it is important to consider the cultural and linguistic environment, for example the inherently stressful nature of a hearing environment. Hearing staff, particularly those without BSL skills, may remind the deaf individual of past abusive relationships and run the risk of re-traumatising their clients. This can be rated as 'exposure to destabilisers'.

Overall, the HCR-20 and the SVR-20 are useful and can be employed with deaf people cautiously and with caveats. However, additional risks relating to deafness, identified by the clinical team, should be incorporated into the assessment and the status of the measure in relation to deaf people be made explicit in the report.

PSYCHOPATHY CHECKLIST–REVISED (PCL-R)

The PCL-R (Hare, 1991) is seen as the gold standard in the measurement of psychopathy. Psychopathy can be conceptualised as an extreme representation of personality disorder. An enduring and inflexible pattern, it is linked with distress for the individual and those around her or him. Psychopathy affects cognition, affective patterns, interpersonal functioning and impulse control.

Research from the US and UK has shown that violent offenders with a high score on the PCL-R are three times more likely to offend than other violent offenders without such a score (Quinsey *et al.*, 1995).

Best practice dictates that administration of the PCL-R is undertaken by two trained individuals who review the information on file, drawing out static risk factors, and then conduct a lengthy semi-structured interview with the individual concerned. Each clinician rates all items separately and records the justification for the score given. Scores are compared and significant differences discussed and resolved.

The PCL-R rates the individual on two factors and four facets. The factors relate to personality traits associated with psychopathy and behavioural characteristics, such as criminal versatility, poor behavioural controls and juvenile delinquency.

In rating collateral information from files, the same difficulties exist as described above; the quality of the information may be dubious and there may be a history of unreliable diagnoses. With regard to the clinical interview, the aim is to acquire additional information, but also to rate aspects of personality, according to definitions given in the manual. Such traits as 'glibness and superficial charm' and 'callousness' or 'lack of empathy' may be difficult to rate in deaf individuals, and practically impossible when using an interpreter. Research with hearing individuals has established the test/retest and inter-rater reliability of this procedure. However, the equivalent research has not been carried out with deaf people. Furthermore, the issue of validity of items has not been resolved. Characteristics of lack of empathy or callousness that are due to impoverished learning associated with deafness would seem, at least at a theoretical level, to be qualitatively different from true psychopathic traits.

Despite its status in risk research, or maybe because of it, the use of the PCL-R is not recommended for deaf people. Whereas the HCR-20 can be seen as aiding the clinician in producing an informed structured clinical judgement, the PCL-R produces a score and a cut-off point. A high score can be extremely damning for an individual as it is linked with individuals who are difficult to engage and often deemed 'untreatable'. It would be unwise to use such a powerful tool with deaf people in the absence of research establishing its validity and reliability and without a protocol for conducting the interview and rating aspects of personality.

RISK OF SEXUAL VIOLENCE PROTOCOL (RSVP)

The RSVP (Hart *et al.*, 2003) is a fairly new means of structured clinical judgement, relating to sexual violence, which takes risk management further than previously. It takes a similar approach to the instruments discussed above, combining a static and dynamic risk factors and a consideration of the environment in which risk might occur. However, each item is rated for past, present or future relevance. In addition, having considered the risk items, there is the opportunity for multidisciplinary discussion of possible future risk scenarios. This allows for deafness-specific factors to be built into the assessment in relation to the person and a variety of settings in which a person might find themselves.

Although, as with other measures, there is no research validating the use of this instrument with deaf people, clinically it has proved very useful in focusing the clinical team on several issues relevant to risk at the same time.

BEST PRACTICE IN RISK ASSESSMENT WITH DEAF PEOPLE

The ideal of a specialist risk assessment may not always be possible; a deaf person in prison or in a hearing service without access to specialists still requires risk assessment. In this situation, a non-specialist professional should always seek advice and supervision from a specialist in forensic mental health and deafness as well as employing a registered qualified interpreter with experience in mental health and deafness. A useful addition to the assessment is the employment of a relay. This is a deaf individual who can take the interpreted version of a question and be creative in how this is communicated to the deaf person. Although this is recommended, particularly when the person being assessed has minimal language skills, it has to be noted that the addition of more people to the assessment process may alter the question and the responses and thus reduce reliability. This would not necessarily be problematic, except that the non-signing clinician is in the dark, left with the impression that what he or she has asked is what is being interpreted. In this situation, there is no issue of negligence or incompetence on the part of the interpreter or relay; on the contrary, they are doing what is required in order to deliver the message in a way the deaf person will understand. However, a dialogue between clinician, interpreter and relay is useful in order that the clinician becomes aware of the changes in language which are taking place in the interpretation process.

Finally, although instruments such as the HCR-20 can be used, reports should make clear the limitations and uncertainties that exist when using these measures with deaf people.

WORKING TO REDUCE RISK

FACILITATING AN UNDERSTANDING OF RISK

For those with impoverished life experiences, or minimal language skills, 'risk' can be a difficult concept to convey. Synonymous with 'danger', the individual may be very resistant to the discussion of risk, as they feel the clinician is saying they are dangerous, which implies something intrinsic about their personality. Understanding that risk can increase and decrease is crucial in therapeutic work; there is a danger that the individual learns the sign 'risk' with no real understanding.

Where there are difficulties in understanding, it is preferable to avoid using the sign 'risk' at first. Beginning by discussing past behaviours, the clinician can start to introduce the idea that certain factors mean such behaviour will definitely happen or might happen or definitely will not happen, perhaps on a sliding scale:

0_____5_____10

Will not happen	May happen	Will happen

Introducing the idea of possibilities can be difficult, as some people can only talk about what is within their direct experience and not conditional propositions. However, the more visual this can be made, the better.

In collaborating with the patient in a discussion of risk, the assessment become less of an exercise done by professionals to the deaf person and more of a joint venture in which the deaf person can experience some feelings of mastery over their future. The tendency to 'fake good' in order to secure a discharge is likely to be decreased if the patients feel they have some contribution to make to risk management, which is taken seriously by the clinical team.

PSYCHOEDUCATIONAL INTERVENTION

Psychoeducational intervention involves the acquisition or practice of skills, and is often delivered in a group setting. Such groups may involve thinking skills, problem-solving, social-skills teaching or anxiety management. Although not directly addressing offending behaviours, pychoeducational work can impact positively on risk in a number of ways.

A characteristic of many deaf offenders who commit violent acts is the inability to think of alternative responses. Interventions use psychological means to teach alternative ways of behaving in a given situation and allow for a rehearsal of new skills in a safe environment.

In addition, the learning of new skills can give added confidence and reduce the tendency of an individual to act aggressively, because they simply feel better about themselves and more in control of themselves and their environment.

OFFENCE-RELATED WORK AND THERAPY

Offence-related work is specifically targeted at risk and may include sex offender treatment, substance misuse work or interventions aimed at helping the person manage their anger and reduce aggression. Individual or group work is possible, although, given the small number of deaf offenders, organising a reasonably homogeneous group in terms of offence type, communication and ability is always a challenge.

Interventions require adaptation not only in terms of language and presentation but also in terms of content, often requiring a larger educational component than in a hearing group due to the background knowledge required for the group not having been learnt earlier in life. Examples include sex offender work requiring an initial sex education component, a substance misuse group digressing onto general information about brain function in order to look at the effects of substances on the central nervous system.

In terms of delivery of offence-related treatment, packages developed for hearing offenders tend to be heavy with English jargon. For example, in the case of substance misuse, terms such as 'tolerance', 'dependence', 'withdrawal' and 'problem of immediate gratification' are not in common usage. However, with a group of hearing patients, these concepts are relatively straightforward to explain. The task with a group of deaf people is to find a way of explaining the concept in a way that makes sense in BSL. This sometimes takes a long time, lots of examples, role play, drawing and so on. On these occasions, co-working with deaf staff is invaluable as this gives a guide to what works.

Finally, psychotherapy can be seen as a means of reducing risk, particularly in instances where behaviour is linked to past trauma. Trauma may be related to past abuses or to offences and may need to be dealt with prior to offence work to avoid dissociation or re-traumatisation.

When working with deaf patients in therapy, the therapist obviously needs to be fluent in BSL and knowledgeable about Deaf issues.

WHEN PEOPLE DO NOT CHANGE

When offenders are admitted to a mental health facility, there is an expectation that they will change and that risk will be reduced. In some cases, that simply does not happen, in which case clinicians often go to greater and more creative lengths to deliver the treatment, all to no avail. Worse still, there can be an assumption that because an offender has attended treatment they are de facto 'treated' and the risk reduced.

In many cases, the individual is blamed for not changing when in fact they cannot change; what is being asked of them is beyond their ability. This applies particularly to individuals with an organic component to their difficulties, either due to the aetiology of their deafness or some traumatic brain injury. The resulting cognitive impairments are such that the person does not learn from being told, cannot generalise from one situation to another; appears rigid and literal in their thinking and tends to be impulsive. Other individuals with a learning disability are not able to benefit from treatment to the extent that risk will be reduced sufficiently to allow community living. When this is the case, it is important that there is acknowledgement within the clinical team that the person concerned can only make limited progress and that this is not their fault or a matter of lack of cooperation or commitment. Long-term plans for an external management of risk via supervision might be necessary. Intervention then becomes a matter of rehabilitation and improving quality of life within the constraints dictated by risk assessment. In other words, there needs to be a conceptual shift away from expecting the individual to change and towards changing the environment and providing the necessary adaptation.

CONCLUSION

Risk assessment of deaf people is a risky business (O'Rourke and Grewer, 2005b) with many pitfalls, which are likely to reduce the reliability and validity of the process. Structured clinical judgement represents best practice in risk assessment of deaf or hearing people. In the case of a deaf person, this should ideally be undertaken by a clinical or forensic psychologist with a knowledge of deaf issues, forensic mental health and deafness and who is fluent in BSL. In addition, consultation with the wider clinical team enables additional information and views to be taken into account.

The lesson from tragedies that have led to inquiries is that all the agencies involved in a person's care need to communicate with each other in order to consider risk in a comprehensive manner. Each agency or clinician involved has a piece of the jigsaw or a particular experience of the individual concerned, and these need to be brought together and discussed. In the case of deaf people, this involves a consideration of issues that are particularly relevant in the context of deafness and the Deaf community.

Risk assessment is pointless without risk management, which involves an individualised approach to intervention, taking into account the cultural and linguistic needs of the person. However, not everyone can make the necessary changes and it is sometimes the staff and the environment that need to adapt in order that the deaf person can live as full a life as possible without putting others at risk.

REFERENCES

Boer DP, Hart SD, Kropp PR, Webster CD (1997) *Manual for the Sexual Violence Risk-20*, Vancouver, British Columbia Institute Against Family Violence.

Department of Health and Welsh Office (1999) *Code of Practice: Mental Health Act (1983)*, London, TSO.

Gardner W, Lidz CW, Mulvey EP, Shaw EC (1996) Clinical versus actuarial predictions of violence in patients with mental illness. *Journal of Consulting and Clinical Psychology* 64(3): 602–9.

Gregory S (1978) *Deaf Children and their Families*, Cambridge, Cambridge University Press.

Hanson RK, Thornton D (1999) *Static-99: Improving Actuarial Risk Assessment for Sex Offenders*, Ottawa, Department of the Solicitor General of Canada.

Hare RD (1991) *Manual for the Hare Psychopathy Checklist–Revised*, Toronto, Multi-Health Systems.

Harris GT, Rice ME, Quinsey VL (1993) Violent recidivism of mentally disordered offenders: the development of a statistical prediction instrument. *Criminal Justice and Behaviour* 20(4): 315–35.

Hart SD, Kropp PR, Laws DR, Klaver J (2003) *The Risk of Sexual Violence Protocol*, Mental Health, Law and Policy Institute, Simon Fraser University.

Hindley P (1997) Psychiatric aspects of hearing impairment. *Journal of Child Psychiatry* 38(1): 101–17.

O'Rourke S, Gahir M, Reed R, Richardson S *et al.* (2005a) *Prison Scoping Exercise*, Report to the Department of Health, unpublished document.

O'Rourke S, Grewer G (2005b) Assessment of deaf people in forensic mental health settings: a risky business! *Journal of Forensic Psychiatry and Psychology* 16(4): 671–84.

Quinsey V, Rice ME, Harris GT (1995) Actuarial prediction of sexual recidivism. *Journal of Interpersonal Violence* 10(11): 85–105.

Vernon M, Rich S (1997) Pedophilia and deafness. *American Annals of the Deaf* 142(4): 300–10.

Webster CD, Douglas KS, Eaves D, Hart SD (1997) *HCR-20 Assessing Risk for Violence, Version 2*, British Columbia, Mental Health, Law and Policy Institute, Simon Fraser University.

Young A, Howarth P, Ridgeway S, Monteiro B (2001) Forensic referrals to the three specialist psychiatric units for deaf people in the UK. *Journal of Forensic Psychiatry* 12(1): 19–35.

Young A, Monteiro B, Ridgeway S (2000) Deaf people with mental health needs in the criminal justice system: a review of the UK literature. *Journal of Forensic Psychiatry* 11(3): 556–70.

Index

Deafness and Challenging Behaviour: The 360° Perspective. Edited by S. Austen and D. Jeffery
© 2007 John Wiley & Sons Ltd